Elastic Habits

How to Create Smarter Habits That Adapt to Your Day

By
Stephen Guise

Blog: stephenguise.com

Book site: minihabits.com

Copyright & Disclaimer

Elastic Habits by Stephen Guise

Contents

INTRODUCTION

"What we do now echoes in eternity."

— Marcus Aurelius

Nobody follows the exact paths they expect to take in life. Being detoured against our will is the rule, not the exception. In such a life of change, obstacles, pain, and surprises, our habits are there for us. By developing and practicing good habits each day, you affirm that you *do* have control over the very core of your life in the midst of the chaos.

Many people understand the importance of friends and family for external support, but not as many recognize the importance of their habits for internal support. Even with world class external support, many still fall into despair because they lack internal support.

Nobody else can live your life for you, no matter how much they love you.

Healthy habitual behaviors stabilize us in stressful times. If you don't have a habitual base of self-supporting behaviors, what do you think happens when your world is rocked? Habits are known wins, and a distressed mind wants and needs nothing more than a known win. If you don't have an internal foundation of good habits, then you will seek the only thing within your reach—bad habits.

Whereas good habits help us recover from hard times, bad habits can deepen negative spirals. This is as blunt as it is important: *habits are the most leveraged aspect of our lives, and we get to choose them.*

1

Better Than Mini Habits

When I finished writing my first book, *Mini Habits,* in 2013, I predicted that it would be successful, purely on the strength of the strategy. I was right, as it became an international bestseller in 17 languages.

Mini Habits has changed thousands of lives all over the world. Six years later, this book and its strategy are even better. I don't mean it in an incremental sense, like with my second and third books. *Elastic Habits* takes a bigger step forward for habit formation than *Mini Habits,* not necessarily because it is more revolutionary (though it may be), but because it is *complete.*

You're going to encounter ideas, physical tools, and strategies in this book that you never have encountered before. If mini habits are fun, rewarding, and effective, then elastic habits are *super* fun, *extra* rewarding, and paradigm-shifting. *Elastic Habits* is more than the evolution of *Mini Habits*: it re-thinks how to approach habits. It takes the base strategy of *Mini Habits*, maintaining all of its proven benefits, and adds the superpower of elasticity. I'm so excited to tell you more, but first, let me tell you about the experiment I did to test this strategy.

The Slump

Since I was a kid, I've been on the "I'll just watch the movie" end of the work ethic spectrum. Whether it was from birth (nature) or video game training (nurture Halo 3), I did *not* like to work. Thus, I'm a different type of author from the ones people are used to reading in this genre. I'm not some super-elite achiever telling people how they can be awesome just like me (!).

It would be generous to say I have an average work ethic, even now. But what I lack in work ethic, I make up for by using the very best strategies. The nice thing about winning strategies is that they help "lazy" people like me *and* natural world-beaters alike. Great strategies are scalable to all levels. As such, the strategies in this book can benefit anyone, whether they're at the top of the proverbial mountain, at rock bottom, or somewhere in between.

About the time I graduated high school, I gained interest in doing something useful with my life. What a pesky internal conflict that turned out to be! With my lazy disposition and bad habits, I struggled to take useful actions. My entire teenage body resisted productivity, as if doing my homework would irreparably harm me. My desire to become someone greater outmatched my behavioral capacity to do so, causing significant frustration and inner angst. I needed answers.

First, I ran into the typical "get motivated" and "just do it" advice. It didn't work for me. Setting normal goals didn't work. My only reliable skill, it seemed, was finding an excuse to quit before I made meaningful progress in areas that mattered to me. I knew what I needed to do, but couldn't get myself to do it. I *still* needed answers.

After 10 years of mostly running in place, I stumbled upon the mini habits idea, which changed my behavior and my life. I finally found a strategy to take me where I wanted to go. After my success with the strategy, I excitedly wrote the *Mini Habits* book to share it with others.

Five years later, I had the idea for elastic habits. I had done well with mini habits, but one day I asked myself why my daily goal always had to be the same. Why couldn't my goals morph to match my needs each day? I wanted to explore this idea, but there was a problem.

I had already formed good habits with *Mini Habits*, and those once-elusive behaviors had become easy to do. That's the beauty of habit! But I had a new idea to test (this book), and I wanted to know if it could help me, even if I was at rock bottom. I was doing well, so I needed to wreck my life to find out.

When others were making the New Year's Resolutions that were destined to fail a month later, I decided to do the opposite. I would *purposely fail* for a month and a half to start the year, and then (try to) emerge from it like a dragon out of a volcano. I called it "the slump." It worked. Good or bad habits won't go away permanently, but by abstaining from them for a month or two, they will go dormant from lack of activation. Mine sure did.

45 Days of Misery
I stopped exercising. I ate unhealthy food. I drank *a lot* more alcohol than usual. I gambled at local casinos frequently and stayed up late. I spent most of every day on the couch watching TV. In many ways, I lived the opposite life of the one I wanted. I indulged in every craving, and said no to every inclination to invest in myself.

The mental side effects were shocking, and worse than I expected. It didn't take long for me to start thinking terrible things about who I was and how little I was worth. Even though I knew this was a purposeful and temporary experiment, it didn't matter. The more you do something, the more it defines you.

After just three weeks, I felt defeated. Hope was gone. The slump had penetrated my *soul*. It saddened me to think of how many others have spiraled into and from this position. Once your spirit breaks, it's shocking how easy it is to decline.

Here's what happened to me physically: I gained 10 pounds of fat, something I had never done before in my life, let alone in a single month. I couldn't sleep. My back was tight and spasmed constantly from poor couch posture. I had debilitating tension headaches and had to go to urgent care three times.

Most surprising of all, I was the most stressed out I've ever been in my life. Both of my eyelids twitched constantly (which continued for months). Doing nothing is somehow the *most* stressful lifestyle. I felt as if I would die if I did this much longer. Inactivity, poor sleep, and poor nutrition were a three-headed monster that drained my vigor; my brain and body seemed to erode at the cellular level.

I purposely "slumped" to become a lethargic, depressed, unmotivated, sickly person. Mission accomplished (sad face). Emotionally, I was in a bad place. Physically, I was in a bad place. It wasn't fun.

After living on the couch for more than a month, even light exercise was daunting. It's not always the lack of desire that stops us (I wanted to exercise); sometimes it's the lack of hope, belief, and self-trust that saps our energy and convinces us we can't do it. I felt that. I wasn't sure I'd *be able* to exercise once my slump ended.

From this experiment, it was clear to me why the people who most *need* to change are often the ones who most struggle to do it. After the experiment, I felt overwhelmed and incapable of change. I genuinely wondered if I had fallen too far. The weight of all the work I knew I needed to do to get back to my normal self (let alone grow further) was on my slumped, stress-tightened shoulders.

You might think I'm embellishing this story, but take a moment to consider the actual impact of not taking care of yourself for 45 days in a row. *It's rough.* I had the freedom to stay home and really let myself go, leaning into self-destruction. The negative impact of poor living compounds daily in much the same way that good habits do, only for the worse. I was a shell of myself, weak in every sense of the word.[1]

The Recovery

I broke out of the slump successfully using the strategies and tools in this book. The elasticity of my habits helped me mend my broken wings at a slow, flexible pace. It gave me the opportunity to try flying at full speed on any given day. *It supported me without insulting my potential, a rare but inspiring combination.*

Even when I couldn't fly as high as I wished, I still achieved victory every day. As these victories began to stack, I started to remember where I was, *who I was*, before I started the slump.

While the slump took a toll on me—thank God my eyelids *finally* stopped twitching and my back has recovered—the experience confirmed that the strategy I'm about to share with you is the real deal. Not only did I come out of the slump successfully, but in the second month of my "dragon out of the volcano" recovery plan, I began eclipsing what I had *ever* accomplished in my five years with *Mini Habits* (and *that* transformation itself was massive!). I continue to soar to even greater heights with my elastic habits, and very soon, you can too.

Be a Soaring Bird

We've made a false assumption about our personal growth —that it's all up to us. It's up to us to get motivated to do what matters. It's up to us to find the will to create positive change in our lives. We assume (and are told) that success is born from heroic effort, but don't ever tell that to a soaring bird.

Most birds maintain flight by flapping their wings to create lift. A relatively small subset of birds know of a better way. *Soaring birds* can fly and even gain elevation by holding their outstretched wings in place. Common soaring birds that you may have seen include seagulls, hawks, pelicans, eagles, and vultures.

There are two environmental phenomena that allow soaring birds to fly without flapping their wings: thermals and updrafts.

Updrafts happen commonly at mountain ridges. When wind hits the side of a ridge, the air has nowhere to go but up. This rising air under the wings of a soaring bird is enough to maintain or increase their elevation.

Thermals are pockets of air a couple of degrees warmer (or more) than the surrounding air. We've all heard that heat rises, and this is the case with thermals, as they are columns of warm(er), rising air. They, too, can support a soaring bird.

Any time you see a bird flying in a circular pattern without flapping its wings, you can be assured that it is a soaring bird and has found a thermal. The bird can circle around the column of air, effortlessly gliding higher and higher. Audubon, a non-profit organization dedicated to protecting birds, says, "Thermal riding requires precise body positioning to stay in the sweet spots that let vultures and all other raptors soar without flapping—a debilitating energy drain."[2]

By using thermals and updrafts, soaring birds rarely have to flap their wings, saving them a lot of energy. These are my kind of birds, because they're possibly lazy, but definitely smart fliers.[3]

We've all tried flapping our proverbial wings to exhaustion before. But have we found the best thermals and updrafts of life? If we can learn to put ourselves in advantageous positions as soaring birds do, we can fly higher in life with *less* effort.

In this book, you'll learn how to...

- Reach the upper heights of your ambition while keeping safe from the downward pressure of gravity.
- Introduce new types and levels of flexibility in your life, allowing you to find the right "motivational thermals" of each unique day.
- Soar with a freedom and weightlessness you've never experienced before.

Let's get started. This book will read as fast as a peregrine falcon.

PART ONE

Death to Rigidity, Long Live Freedom

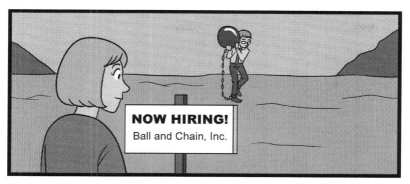

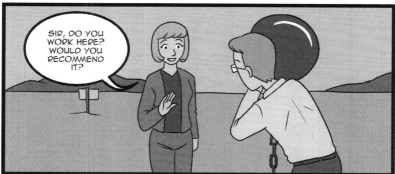

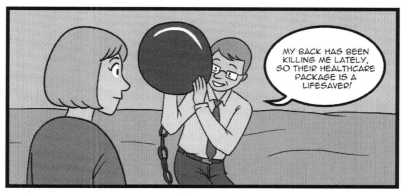

**Freedom is priceless, and always the superior path.
Never sacrifice it for temporary gain.**

Chapter 1
Fluid Lives, Rigid Goals

"Just as water retains no constant shape, so in warfare there are no constant conditions. He who can modify his tactics in relation to his opponent and thereby succeed in winning, may be called a heaven-born captain."

— Sun Tzu

If I asked you to choose one of these three superpowers, which would you choose?

1. The ability to fly.
2. The ability to see one week into the future.
3. The ability to master one skill per day.

I would choose flying just because of how much fun it would be, though the other two options are tempting enough to make me think twice. But you know what I'd really love? A fourth option that would let me choose one of the three options each day. Wouldn't you?

It would be objectively smarter to choose the flexible option. Even if you always chose the same power every day (unlikely), you wouldn't lose anything by having the option to do something else. *It doesn't hurt to have options, and it sure can help.*

Wouldn't it be nice if you could choose whether to fly, know the future, or master new skills, *depending on the exact momentary circumstances of your life*? Those particular superpowers aren't included with this book, but the demonstrated superpower of flexibility is. With elastic habits and goals, you'll be prepared to maximize your potential in all situations. Your daily goals will survive down days, and thrive on others, depending on what's needed and what you want to do.

Most strategies require consistent positivity and high energy to succeed. But this strategy is engineered to work with your thought patterns, whether they're positive, negative, or neutral. It gives you a helping, nonjudgmental hand when you fall down and pushes you higher when you're on your feet and ready to go. Unlike strategies that attempt to control your behavior, this one works *with you and for you*.

If this all sounds nice in theory, you're reading the right book. If it sounds impossibly optimistic, I understand your skepticism, but stay with me. This is the best personal development and habit strategy I've ever used, by far, and I've tried everything.

Daily small commitments are considered by many to be the most effective habit formation strategy, and that's why they've become the standard. But they are only part of what can be a much greater, much more effective strategy.

The Motion of Life

Save for Phil Connors, not one person in the history of the world has ever lived the same day twice. If you live to be 70, that's 25,550 unique, yet interconnected days. Our lives are best described as *fluid*. Each second, minute, hour, and day flows into the next, and it's always in motion, always changing. Like the ocean, life has:

- Sudden highs and lows (just like waves rising and crashing).
- Sustained periods of highs and lows (just like ocean tides).
- Positive and negative momentum across multiple levels of time (just like currents and countercurrents, rip currents, surface currents, and deep currents).
- In-laws (just like bluntnose sixgill sharks).

Like ocean waters, life constantly moves in multiple ways. There are patterns, but it's never completely predictable, and oftentimes surprising. Thus, to be successful in life in the short term and long term, you must be able to thrive in a fluid, ever-changing environment. It's a shame, then, that we don't even try.

For too long, we have set rigid goals, trying to do the exact same action, regardless of the conditions we face. We do it in the name of grit, in the name of consistency and habit formation, or in the name of being courageous or persistent. But here's a real-life, oceanic example of why forcing ourselves to unflinchingly adhere to preset ideas is, well, stupid.

Riptide Regret

Imagine you're in the ocean. You're splashing around, thinking about the possibility of swimming in the same waters as ~~in-laws~~ bluntnose sixgill sharks. Yikes. You decide to head to the beach to sun-dry and read *Elastic Habits*. (This book is self-aware and self-promoting.)

People are watching, you assume, so you decide to show off your beautiful butterfly stroke as you swim in to shore.

After a minute, you stop for a rest, wipe your eyes, pause, and say out loud, "What is this, a beach for ants?"

Gratuitous galloping gazelles! Those aren't ants, they're people! Then you realize ... you're far from the shore because you're caught in a riptide.

To be "courageous, persistent, and strong," you stick with your original plan to swim directly towards the shore with butterfly, the most impressive but most tiring swimming stroke. You strain against the current and gasp for air as your muscles fatigue rapidly. The sea is relentless and you aren't getting any closer. You swim harder and harder until, eventually, exhaustion sets in. You drown.

It's a sad (thankfully fictional) tale with an important lesson. In the story, the situation changed drastically but you, the swimmer, didn't. You started out swimming butterfly to shore to impress your friends and stuck with that plan to your end. But once you realized you were in a rip current, your objective changed from "impress people" to "survive." **When your situation changes your objective, it calls for a new strategy.**

A riptide, or rip current, is a strong but narrow current of water that goes from shore out to sea. People do die in them, and it often works exactly as described above—they panic, swimming furiously and directly into the strength of the current until they're too exhausted to stay afloat.

With a calm mind and smart strategy, however, there are *multiple ways* to escape a rip current. The best option is to swim parallel to the shoreline before swimming towards it.[1] This is a good metaphor for life, since swimming "sideways" doesn't look like progress, but is sometimes a necessary step to make progress. Since rip currents are relatively narrow, it won't take too long to exit it and swim back to shore. The second option is to simply relax and let the current take you out to sea until it dissipates, and call for help (if you need it) swimming back. The main danger comes when you insist on overcoming the rip current by swimming directly into it and exhausting yourself.

Improvisation: The Forgotten Power of the Brain

Humans are uniquely suited to succeed in a variety of circumstances because of our immeasurable ability to adapt and conquer challenges. We're phenomenal problem solvers in real time, with one important caveat. For us to adapt successfully, we must first choose to be adaptable.

Roughly 99.9947% of goal and habit strategies are inflexible. They ask you to *power through* and *do whatever it takes* to meet some arbitrary preselected requirements that can't and don't consider your unique life. They forbid you to improvise. That's a problem the instant you get sick, injured, burned out, exhausted, or have a once-in-a-lifetime opportunity that requires the full day. That kind of stubbornness gets you killed in a rip current; it kills goals and habits, too.

Nothing can replace your brain when it comes to adapting to your environment and making the most of your current situation. Your brain is the key to your success!

When something as dynamic and intelligent as your mind is forced to do one thing, disallowing on-the-fly adjustments in favor of following an arbitrary standard, it's a declaration of war. You know your life, abilities, and limits in real time better than any "one size fits all" program could ever hope to. So, even if a rigid system fits into your life for longer than two weeks, you will eventually rebel on principle and for the sake of freeing your powerful mind.[2]

The idea is not that we must consciously decide everything we do; it's that we can give ourselves *the option* to shift a goal when circumstances call for it. With the freedom to shift habits up, down, or even sideways, winning streaks can extend for *years*, and you can make the most out of any situation. You'll never feel trapped, because your habits will change with you and the circumstances you face.

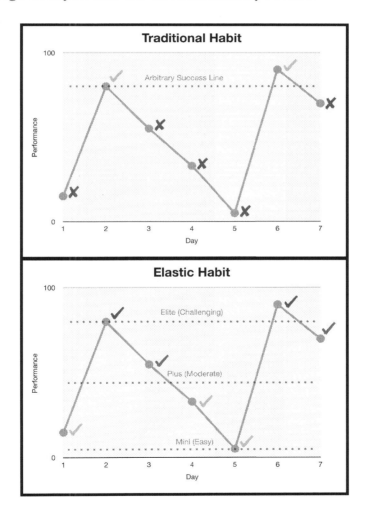

We've assumed that we must find the Goldilocks spot for our habits and goals, the one spot that isn't too easy or too hard, and just rewarding enough. *But that spot moves every day.* Just think a moment about the range of days you've had. On some days, you may feel like conquering the world. On others, you may feel like surviving is an accomplishment in itself. No single goal can satisfy the many situations we face in life.

Chapter 1 Closing Thoughts

Our lives are fluid and volatile. Why do we make our habits rigid and brittle? There must be a better approach.

Elastic Habits theme song plays*

Chapter 2
The Power of Freedom

"They who can give up essential liberty to obtain a little temporary safety deserve neither liberty nor safety."

— Benjamin Franklin

Discipline is not self-discipline.

Growing up, we are disciplined by parents, teachers, and other authorities. If we do something wrong, we're punished. If we do something right, we're rewarded (or at least not punished).

The concept of controlling one's behavior for a particular set of results is familiar by the time we're adults. But our concept of discipline is almost always the externally motivated (discipline) form rather than the internally produced (self-discipline) form. Some are able to internalize discipline into self-discipline, but not everyone does, especially when we gain a surplus of freedom in adulthood. Why is that?

Discipline is driven by external punishment and reward. Self-discipline, however, is driven by freedom and practice.

Freedom Enables Self-Discipline

The paradoxical fog begins to clear once you separate the two ideas. Discipline is what authority figures do *to us* to keep us in check. Self-discipline is what we do *for ourselves* to gain control of our lives and become the people we desire to be.[1]

> "Essentially, [self-discipline] must be encouraged, rather than enforced."
> ~ SiXiong Lester Walters

Self-discipline is a skill, but it's only possible to sustain it through freedom of choice. As strange as it sounds, you cannot force self-discipline upon yourself. You can't say, "I'm self-disciplined from this point onward!" Why? You might not have the skill to sustain it and will *always* have the choice to abort the mission. Always!

You can force action at times, yes, but *self-discipline isn't a one-time choice*, it's a practiced skill. Just as playing guitar once doesn't make you a guitar player, forcing yourself to abstain from chocolate or go to the gym one time doesn't make you self-disciplined.

If we put together all the information we've covered thus far in the book, about goals, life, freedom, discipline, and self-discipline, it explains why so many people struggle to control their behavior. Point by point, see if you agree with these statements:

1. Life is fluid, unpredictable, and always changing with highs, lows, and sixgill sharks.
2. The human brain is powerful, dynamic, and adept at problem solving, making it well suited to improvise in response to life's changing conditions.
3. Most goals and systems are rigid, unadaptable, and seemingly oblivious to the nature of life, which can make our powerful and capable brains feel like

prisoners.
4. Discipline is what others do to us to keep our behavior in check.
5. Self-discipline is how we form ourselves into the people we want to be.

When you put everything together, do you see the issue?

People model their change attempts after the external discipline they receive as children. They try to improve their lives by enslaving themselves to rigid and arbitrary goals, an outside-in approach. But for real change to occur, we need self-discipline, which can *only* come from a place of personal freedom and empowerment. We need to do the opposite of what we typically do.

- We set up harsh, rigid objectives as an attempt to simulate that external punishing force: *I will do 100 push-ups every single day.* Instead, we can have flexible goals.
- We raise expectations and stakes: *I must do this, no matter what. No excuses.* Instead, we can situationally adjust expectations and stakes.
- We punish ourselves for noncompliance: *If I don't do this, I am a failure and should be ashamed of myself.* Instead, we can encourage all progress and eliminate shame, which only weakens the self and one's sense of freedom.

Say No to Self-Slavery
It's not rotten to force yourself to do good things sometimes. But it's often taken to the level of self-slavery, where you feel like a prisoner to your plans instead of the commander of your life. Self-slavery happens as a result of confusing the appearance of self-discipline with the actual mechanism behind it. Self-discipline often looks like self-

slavery to the untrained eye, but real self-discipline is a labor of love born from freedom.

If changing your behavior has always felt like a struggle and a burden, ask yourself why. What's more satisfying than living how you want to live? What's more important than pursuing your values? What's more exciting than becoming and being the person you want to be? Behavior change can be hard work and requires patience, no doubt, but if done correctly, it's joyful, fun, freeing work.

You need to like and respect what you're doing (and all it entails) if you want to keep doing it for weeks, months, and years. That means you can't feel like a slave to your goals; you must feel like—and be—the master. What do slaves always want? Freedom from whatever enslaves them. You'll quit anything that resembles bondage, as you should. Self-discipline is freedom, and if cultivated correctly, it will feel that way too.

There's no supernatural force preventing us from living our best lives. We tend to stop ourselves. Here's why: Those who trade their freedom for temporary results will inevitably trade it back later because freedom matters most to us. Those who act with freedom from the start have no reason to stop themselves.

The crux of my argument comes down to this: Action birthed from freedom is more powerful and effective than action birthed from brute force. The only possible argument for forced action is that, while it's uncomfortable at times, at least it's effective. But those who believe that are underestimating the power of freedom.

Freedom is the only path worth considering, because if freedom is innately more important to us than nearly anything else, we can't afford to sacrifice it for the sake of our goals. Sadly, we often do sacrifice freedom for short-term gain. Instead, we can leverage freedom's power to pursue our goals.

Liberty or Death

"Why stand we here idle? What is it that gentlemen wish? What would they have? Is life so dear or peace so sweet as to be purchased at the price of chains and slavery? Forbid it, Almighty God—I know not what course others may take; but as for me—give me liberty or give me death!"

~ Patrick Henry

If we can agree that freedom is powerful,[2] the question becomes: What role does it play in habit and goal pursuit?

Is Freedom Ever Bad?

One could look at my slump and say, "Look at what the freedom to indulge did to you!" But that wasn't freedom, it was slavery to indulgent living, since I forbade most of my good habits. It was the same kind of arbitrary restriction or requirement that goal-setters place upon themselves.

That being said, I understand that some may use their freedom to choose "the slump lifestyle." I've done it before. It's no wonder, then, that we are so quick to sacrifice our freedom, which carries risk and uncertainty. We like certainty.

Freedom is like a table saw. You can make a nice cabinet with it, but you can also cut your finger off. Skill and strategy determine whether you add a cabinet or subtract a finger. We need a systematic way to use the saw's power without putting our digits at risk.

Because freedom is powerful, it must be paired with practice. If given the absolute freedom *and ability* to do whatever we want, of course most of us will use our freedom for our own good. Freedom gives us the power, and practice gives us the skill. This book provides the framework and strategy that enable safe daily practice through freedom.

Freedom scares us because it amplifies who we really are. For example, people fear that allowing themselves to eat whatever they want will result in bingeing and weight gain, so they restrict themselves and go on a diet. *But, as I covered extensively in Mini Habits for Weight Loss, studies show that dieters binge more and gain more weight than non-dieters.* It sounds surprising, until you consider that dieters are slaves to their chosen diet. What do slaves do? They rebel. They seek freedom. Lesson: Don't make a cheeseburger the symbol of freedom if you want to lose weight.

Next, we'll explore elasticity and how it gives you freedom to naturally build habits to fit your unique life. It changes everything you've ever been taught about pursuing goals and forming habits.

Chapter 2 Closing Thoughts

To be human is to desire the freedom to live in your own way. Some temporarily trade their freedom for short-lived results (dieting, for example), but those who protect and leverage their freedom can make the greatest leaps forward and sustain those changes.

PART TWO

Elasticity and Flexibility

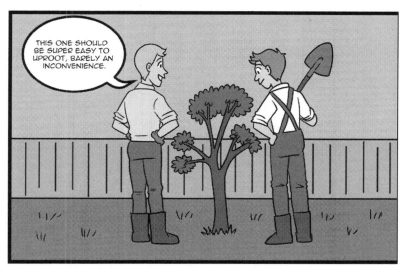

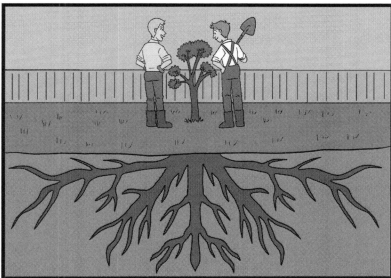

When one root fails, the others provide support.
Flexibility is the ultimate source of strength.

Chapter 3
Flexibility Is Strength

"Water is fluid, soft, and yielding. But water will wear away rock, which is rigid and cannot yield. As a rule, whatever is fluid, soft, and yielding will overcome whatever is rigid and hard. This is another paradox: what is soft is strong."

— Lao Tzu

Here is the definition of *elasticity*,[1] according to Merriam-Webster dictionary:

Elasticity (n): the quality or state of being elastic: such as
  A. the capability of a strained body to recover its size and shape after deformation
  B. RESILIENCE (physics, see below)
  C. the quality of being adaptable

As for which of these definitions relates to the strategies in this book, the answer is *all of them and more.*

Elasticity in Physics
One of the best synonyms for *elastic* is *resilient*. It aptly describes each way in which a material's elasticity can be measured.

In physics, there is the *elastic limit*, or the amount a

material can stretch until it is *permanently* deformed. If a material is stretched and is able to snap back to its original shape, it has not yet reached its elastic limit. Pull a little bit on a rubber band, and it will stretch before returning to its original shape. If the rubber band is stretched and loosens (or breaks), then it has surpassed its elastic limit.

An *elastic modulus* is a measure of a material's resistance to temporary deformation when a stress is applied to it. So, in the case of a rubber band, its elastic limit is relatively high, but its elastic modulus is low since it's easily (temporarily) deformed. In the case of a diamond, its elastic modulus is high since it is very resistant to denting, breaking, bending, and stretching. The fact that elasticity can be looked at in two different ways is very meta of it. Even the term itself is flexible!

While it may seem strange for these different aspects of elasticity to coexist in physics, consider that they measure the same thing, just in different ways—resilience against pressure. Diamond resists pressure by being the hardest natural substance on Earth and not giving in to it. Rubber resists pressure by *giving into it* and changing shape to "accommodate" the pressure, before ultimately springing back to its original shape. Once pressure is removed from these elastic materials, they remain just as they started (if the force was below their elastic limits). In both cases, the materials are resilient, not changing as a result of applied pressure.

Grasping the full meaning of elasticity helps us to see its true benefit. Elasticity is not only about increasing flexibility; it's about increasing resilience to pressure. For anyone wanting to form habits, that idea should resonate immediately. Wouldn't you like your goals and habits to be resilient under pressure so that they can withstand challenges, last longer, and improve your life? You can do so by making them more elastic.

Why Flexibility Is Strength

This book is called *Elastic Habits*, so it shouldn't be too surprising that we're discussing flexibility. What may be surprising, however, is the idea that flexibility itself can be a source of world-class strength. Here are four reasons why flexibility can provide strength and resilience:

1. Multiple roots are better than one.

One of my favorite movie scenes is in *The Lord of the Rings: The Two Towers.* In the city of Isengard, the evil wizard Sarumon is seen building an Orc army in an underground factory, which is fueled by burning nearby trees. The Ents are massive tree beings that can walk and talk, and, being trees, they decide to fight for their wooden brothers and sisters. They attack Isengard.

In addition to crushing, kicking, and otherwise dismantling Orcs with their powerful branch-limbs, the Ents break a massive dam nearby. Then, to prevent themselves being upended by rushing waters, they "put down roots" and hold steady. Water destroys the factory and sweeps everything away except for the Ents, who remain rooted to the ground and upright.[2]

Have you ever tried to pull a tree out of the ground? People use chainsaws to cut trees down at the base, because pulling them out by the roots is *not* easy to do, even for a small, non-Ent tree. While a tree trunk is often relatively tall and thin, its sprawling roots give it a wide and stable base. And if one root dies, the other roots are there to support the tree. In addition to increased strength, multiple roots give trees a larger footprint to drink water from, which helps in drier times. Roots are great.

Those without flexibility depend on *one root* to do the job, whatever it may be. One root works great ... until it dies. Multiple roots keep people and trees alike grounded, strong, and far more resilient to adversity.

2. Flexibility enables improvisation.

Improvisation is key in all areas of life because we cannot fully control our environment or what others do. Those who live rigidly will eventually be broken by circumstances they did not want or expect. Those with flexibility can dodge one obstacle, cut through a second roadblock with a diamond-chained chainsaw, rubber-band-slingshot themselves over that pesky third barrier, and change direction well in advance of the fourth.

By embracing flexibility, you will find more ways to succeed through improvisation. The more you're able to improvise, the more proactive and resilient you will be in a random basket of positive and negative circumstances (and consider that "a random basket of positive and negative circumstances" is an apt description of life).

3. Flexibility opens your eyes to opportunities.

Flexibility helps us to maximize opportunities (think more roots to reach more water sources). Additionally, flexibility helps us to *see* more opportunities.

> "All fixed set patterns are incapable of adaptability or pliability. The truth is outside of all fixed patterns."
> ~ Bruce Lee

A fixed mind has only one way of thinking about or doing something, and is blind to all else. While that one thing can be good in certain situations (plowing straight ahead works sometimes), it can be lethal in others. For example, Blockbuster should have pivoted or bought Netflix.

Blockbuster began as a movie rental store in 1985; in 2010, they filed for bankruptcy *as the same movie rental company.* For the first part of their 25 years, brick-and-mortar movie rental was an effective business model. Then, suddenly, video streaming became viable and that business model didn't work anymore. Their one root died and took their entire business down with it. They failed to see other options in time, including the option to buy a small startup called Netflix.

Netflix started out as a movie-mailing service, a novel idea that disrupted Blockbuster's business. They added online streaming in 2007, which became their core business. Fast forward to 2019, and they're a major production company, making numerous TV shows and movies. Their continuous mental and tactical flexibility has made them a market leader in a highly competitive space and one of the best performing stocks of the 21st century (NFLX stock gained over 31,000% from their IPO in 2002 to 2019).

If you have flexibility in your arsenal from the start, you will gain a wider field of vision to better anticipate incoming threats *and* opportunities in your life. You will have multiple tools for different occasions. This doesn't mean you won't have a favorite, go-to tool, only that you'll have (and find) more and better tools to use. Flexibility creates more favorable outcomes through mental dexterity, regardless of whether your current situation is positive or negative.

4. Flexibility lets you allocate resources more efficiently and boosts your sense of freedom.

If you have flexibility as a core part of your strategy, you can flex and bend your goals to whatever suits you best on that day. That means less arbitrary and inefficient task switching for the sake of "following the plan."

As all writers know, in certain magical moments, the words flow well. To that, I say, "Write while the ~~pen~~ keyboard is hot!" Having the flexibility to load up on one behavior on any given day is the ultimate freedom and keeps you motivated to pursue *all* of your goals.

Chapter 3 Closing Thoughts

Flexibility is the most powerful form of resilience against whatever threatens your progress, making it a primary source of strength. With flexibility, you can overcome different types of challenges in multiple ways. In the next chapter, you'll see how vertical and lateral flexibility creates invincible habits.

Chapter 4
A New Dimension of Flexibility

"All men can see the tactics whereby I conquer, but what none can see is the strategy out of which victory is evolved. Do not repeat the tactics which have gained you one victory, but let your methods be regulated by the infinite variety of circumstances."

— Sun Tzu

Mini habits are exceptionally small behaviors done every day to form habits over time. I call them "stupid small" behaviors because they really do sound stupid—painting or drawing for one minute, doing one push-up, or cleaning one corner of a room, for example. Mini habits are deceptively powerful because they are not a ceiling, like most goals, but a floor. You can always do more than your (mini)mum habit, but, importantly, you will always do *something*, which is *infinitely* better than doing nothing.

The Difference between Goals and Habits
I'm going to be talking a lot about goals in this book, but, as the title suggests, this book is about habits. Therefore, I want to explain their connection clearly.

Goals are "an aim or desired result." Habits are "a settled or regular tendency or practice." A goal can be any aim or desired result, including the goal to form a habit. And habits form by completing the same goal each day. You can see the overlap—your long-term goal is to form a habit, which itself is formed by smaller daily goals.

So when I talk about goals, know that I'm talking about *the daily goals that form habits*. To master habit formation, you must master the practice of meeting daily goals consistently. Consistent goal achievement is often thought to be a matter of powering through adversity, but it always starts with making consistency easy.

Many thousands of people across the world have changed their behavior and lives by introducing daily mini habits into their lives. A mini habit, by being "stupid small" and easy to do, automatically prioritizes consistency. Many will claim that consistency is important to them, but when you say, "I must practice guitar for at least two hours per day," you aren't actually prioritizing consistency, you're making consistency more difficult by prioritizing *quantity, ego, rapid results, and achievement.*

To prioritize consistency means to set your marks low enough that you won't ever miss. It means to make your minimum requirement "showing up" instead of "showing off." If you're in any kind of slump (and even if you aren't), a mini habit plan can revitalize you. By showing up every day, you will create spectacular positive forward momentum that builds upon itself exponentially.

So… What's Missing with Mini Habits?

When you look at your goal of doing one sit-up per day, it can feel like something is missing. Sure, it's great to show up and get a small win every day, but at some point soon, you want to see results, progress … *progression to bigger wins.* You want to see evidence that you're really going somewhere with this, that you can make the jump from the mini pond to the ocean.

I don't mean to imply that mini habits alone can't take you to new levels of success—they can and have for many people, including myself. But the *Mini Habits* (or any other) method is not beyond improvement. Case in point: the methods in this book build exponentially upon the existing *Mini Habits* framework.

We're going from mini to elastic because adding flexibility strengthens the strategy in the same way as adding roots strengthens a tree; it will make your daily goals even more resilient, with higher upside potential in the short and long term.

Want Maximum Strength? Get Full Flexibility

You can get strong in a number of ways. But for maximum strength, you need full flexibility. This is true in the human body. If I tried to do a split, it would be hilarious or tragic (depending on your perspective). Gymnasts, however, are disturbingly flexible. Did you know that gymnasts are also, pound for pound, some of the strongest human beings on Earth? Because gymnasts are *flexibly strong*, they even make for good weightlifters, even though they don't specifically train for that.

Gymnastics coach Christopher Sommer said that one of his students was able to deadlift 400 pounds on his first day of high school weight training, despite weighing only 135 pounds! Sommer says, "I've seen many gymnasts capable of planche[1] push-ups do double bodyweight bench presses on their first attempts. Conversely, I've never seen a weightlifter capable of doing a double bodyweight bench press even come close to a planche push-up initially."[2]

Weightlifters tend to train very specific movements and thus become strong in specific ways, but gymnasts train so dynamically that their strength is highly useful in almost all other sports, including weightlifting.

Flexibility is the foundation for ultimate strength.

I didn't include the word "ultimate" there as filler or to sound cool. That's an important distinguishing word, as it's possible to build remarkable strength *without* flexibility. At no point in this book will I suggest that flexibility is the *only* way to become strong or succeed in an area (because, for one, that very statement is inflexible). But I will say that it is the best way, and that *ultimate* strength has to come from a place of flexibility, or else it will merely be *situational strength*.[3]

> "Strength without balance, agility, coordination, and explosiveness is strength that's athletically unusable."
> ~ Christopher Sommer

Now I'll show you how the *Mini Habits* strategy is strong because of its lateral flexibility. Then, I'll introduce the new dimension of flexibility that *Elastic Habits* brings. It's a fun one, and it's fully compatible with your current mini habits if you already have them!

The Mini Habits Weapon: Lateral Flexibility

The *Mini Habits* premise is this: Get the easy win as soon as possible with small daily goals. Once you've won, *then* consider further steps forward. For example, get down and do one push-up. That's much better than zero. Then stop, or do five, 10, or 50 more push-ups if you want.

Mini habits offer excellent *lateral* flexibility. **Lateral flexibility means having a variety of ways to reach a goal, or even the option to change your goal on the fly.** Hybrid mini habits are a good example. These are habits with an either/or win condition—either walk two blocks or do one pull-up to fulfill your exercise habit. The "any time before bed" daily cue brings even more lateral flexibility, as it gives you the entire day to do the habit, instead of forcing you to pick a specific time.

You can complete your mini habit using different cues; you can even complete it in a number of different ways. This flexibility, combined with easy completion, makes it so that you never feel trapped with a mini habit. You can circle around your easy goal and attack it from any angle that suits you each day.

Lateral flexibility is a proven, game-changing weapon that enables remarkable consistency, but lateral flexibility isn't *full* flexibility, is it? If you're playing basketball, you don't only want to move laterally—from side to side and forward and back—you also want up-and-down *verticality*. You want to be able to jump up to dunk or block shots or to dive on the floor for a loose ball.

Maximum strength is only achieved with full flexibility, so we're going to add vertical flexibility to the already successful and laterally flexible *Mini Habits* framework.[4] Let's look at what fully developed vertical flexibility can do.

The New Weapon: Vertical Goal Flexibility
In doing research for this book, I came across something that confirmed what I had suspected for the last few years. I gasped when I found it, because I knew it would have big implications for the future of goal setting and habit pursuit.

A 2017 Stanford study (indirectly) suggested that different goal sizes have inherent strengths and weaknesses.[5]

The study's hypothesis was that different stages of goal pursuit had different (ideal) motivational sources. Let's use the goal of 100 push-ups as an example. The study found that setting a sub-goal of 10 push-ups at a time (instead of the full 100 push-ups) was more effective at motivating people to action at the beginning because it increased their sense of *attainability* (that's a key word we'll discuss in the next chapter). But later on, once people believed they were within reach of the bigger goal, like when they'd already done 75 of 100 push-ups, the sub-goal was *less motivating than the bigger goal.* When they got within striking distance of the bigger picture goal, their strongest source of motivation changed from *attainability* to the *value* to be gained by completing the bigger goal.

This makes sense, doesn't it? The first question we ask is, "Can I actually accomplish this?" But once we see success as inevitable, why focus on small goals when we know we can get the big win?

The researchers at Stanford confirmed their hypothesis over four separate studies. They found different ideal motivational sources at different stages of goal pursuit. This suggests that everyone, myself included, has oversimplified the relationship between motivation and goal pursuit. It suggests that greater strategy is warranted for how we structure our goals.

But I'm taking it a step further. I believe that even the idea of specific and clearly defined "goal stages" is oversimplified to fit the tradition of rigid goal setting (having only one win condition). In reality, it's not a stretch to say that our motivation can change at any time.

I like their proposed general framework of small goals helping us act in the beginning of a pursuit, and goal value encouraging us to finish. But when dealing with habits, there is no finish line. Habits are for life! And yet, in this journey, we still have those periods of belief and doubt.

When we doubt ourselves the most, small goals help us move forward. When we believe in our ability, large goals help us connect to our ultimate vision for success. The same parallels can be said for low and high energy moments, negative and positive emotions, and more. Regardless of what motivational source we need, all we know for sure is that it isn't constant, and that's all we need to know!

If you set only one way to win, then it makes sense that you'd try to fine-tune that win condition to make you as motivated as possible to pursue it. Based on this study, you'd focus on smaller sub-goals in the beginning of your pursuit and the larger goal once you had made significant progress with the small ones. While this is a marked improvement over most strategies, we're going to leap ahead of it, too. Our strategy will not predetermine a single objective. **Full vertical flexibility will allow us to intuitively choose the goal we're most motivated to do today, right now, meaning we don't need to know the exact timing of motivational stages in goal pursuit.**

The nuanced relationship of motivation and goal size has major implications for how we think about and pursue our daily goals and habits for the rest of our lives. I think by looking back on your experience of pursuing differently sized goals, your experience and intuition will chime with what's recently been found in this study.

Different goal sizes have inherent strengths and weaknesses.

Most people would agree that different goal sizes have pros and cons, but it's what we can do with them that's exciting. Let's talk about that, Rhett.

Pies? Pies.

The *Elastic Habits* strategy uses multiple goal sizes to neutralize their weaknesses. From our discussion of flexibility, that idea should make a lot of sense to you, as should the following generalization.

Flexibility creates strength by neutralizing weaknesses.

It's simple. If one root of a tree dies or is cut off, you won't notice when you try to lift it. It will seem (and practically be) just as strong because its strength is diversified over many roots, not just one. Vertical flexibility does the same thing for the daily goals that you intend to turn into lifelong good habits.

How Vertical Flexibility Neutralizes Goal Weaknesses

Vertical flexibility in goal setting means that your goal can increase or decrease in size. To better explain the advantage of this, I'm going to describe two pies, each with three pieces.

One pie will contain the strengths of three primary goal sizes and the other will contain their weaknesses. It's done in this way to show you how the strengths of each goal size fit together to make the perfect "goal pie." Or put into non-stupid terms, this shows how powerful it would be if we could somehow combine the strengths of each goal type into one super-hybrid-mutant goal.

On the flip side, the goal weakness pie contains all of the downsides of goal setting, sorted by goal size. Goal sizes have important-to-know weaknesses too, which is why choosing a goal size is not as simple as picking your favorite strength.

The Goal Strengths Pie
- **Small:** Very easy to start, not intimidating, suitable for remarkable consistency (and building habits), powerful momentum builder.
- **Medium:** Not overly intimidating or difficult to start and moderately satisfying if completed, well-balanced effort/reward ratio.
- **Large:** Can motivate us to "rise to the challenge," aligns with our dreams, impressive and very satisfying if completed, exciting to think about and do.

Wouldn't it be nice if we had access to *all* of those characteristics? Now let's look at the weaknesses.

The Goal Weaknesses Pie
- **Small:** Unimpressive to the point of seeming worthless as individual accomplishments, potentially weak sense of progression if kept small (don't tell *Mini Habits* I said this).
- **Medium:** Fails to get the super-easy starts and consistency benefits of small goals, not as inspiring and satisfying as larger goal wins, seemingly muted benefits compared to the other two sizes.
- **Large:** Often intimidating to the point of paralysis, very difficult to be consistent with (no habit formation soup for you!), demoralizing when you fail or burn out.

The Fallacy of the "Best Goal Size"
As you can see from the pies, there isn't actually a "perfect" goal size. And yet, you have people who swear by each one. This is human nature, isn't it? Pick a slice and fight to the death for it. You see it in politics—more people choose one

side than recognize the merits and flaws of multiple sides. You see it in sports—fans of one team hate the best player(s) on the other team, even though he's won six Super Bowls and is clearly the greatest quarterback of all time. In our quest to find the one "right" answer, we tend to shun the correct parts of other answers while blinding ourselves to the flaws in our own.

Take one more look at the strengths and weaknesses pies. Do you notice anything interesting about them? Do you see the symmetry?

The weakness pie slices are *exactly* countered by the opposite-strength pie slices! For example, the **weakness** of large goals is that they can be intimidating and cause paralysis, and the **strength** of small goals is in *preventing* such intimidation and paralysis. And the primary **weakness** of a small goal has to do with the fact that, on an individual day, we're not going to be all that inspired or excited to practice guitar for one minute. That happens to be the **strength** of a large goal, because it's exciting and inspiring to practice guitar for two hours or master a new song.

The medium goal is right in the middle, balancing out the two extremes. It, too, has benefits and downsides that counter each other. A medium goal isn't amazing, but it isn't small; it's not super-easy, but it's not super hard. It's not the best or the worst. It's in the middle, and *sometimes* that's what we need.

With such a perfectly counterbalanced set of goal sizes, one wonders why we'd ever pick just one and proclaim its strengths while ignoring its weaknesses. Let me repeat the key part of that—**why would we ever pick just one of them?** Why not combine them and find a way to leverage the power of all goal sizes? By doing so, we will neutralize their weaknesses.

If this sounds too good to be true, well, this time it isn't. It's just as good as it sounds! I've done it. I've *lived this*. I was able to emerge from a horrible slump like a lava dragon because of this. This is *full* flexibility for goals and habit formation, fully elastic habits!

The three goal sizes are a specialized team—they each serve a distinct purpose. And you've probably been using only one (as I was)! Or maybe you've been rigidly switching from one to another for long periods of time instead of fluidly switching based on the real-time conditions of your life. No worries. We've all done it before, but your path has brought you to read this book in this moment, which means you have a unique opportunity to live smarter than you ever have before.

The next question: How do we incorporate these three sizes into a system that makes sense, works fluidly, and integrates into our busy lives? We'll cover that in the application chapter.

Right now, we're going to dive into the depths of behavior change and take a look at motivation. I widely criticized motivation in *Mini Habits* because it didn't fit the strategy, but elasticity has changed the game and now motivation plays a big role. We've only touched the surface here, and there are more interesting revelations below. Watch out for the sixgill sharks.

Chapter 4 Closing Thoughts

Goal sizes can work together. Why pick just one when you can gain the power of the whole team?

PART
THREE

Motivation: Unlocked
Through Choice

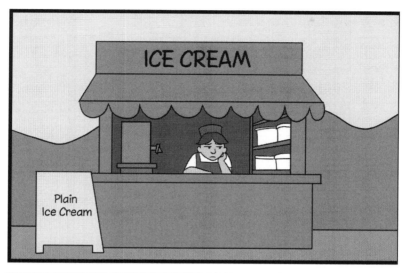

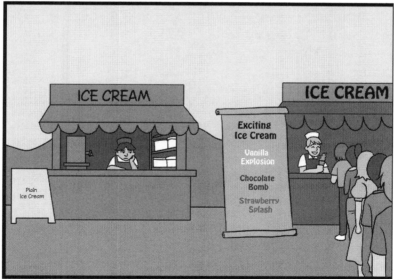

Choice is the spice of life, and a powerful motivator to action.

Chapter 5
A Breakthrough in Motivation

"The pessimist sees difficulty in every opportunity. The optimist sees opportunity in every difficulty."

— Winston Churchill

Motivation drives us to take action. When pursuing a goal or trying to develop good habits, you ideally want to create situations in which your motivation to make progress is relatively high. This might sound strange if you've read *Mini Habits*, since I eschewed motivation in favor of willpower. Here's why it's different now.

Willpower is a conscious decision to act despite not being motivated to act. Willpower remains the best method for doing a mini habit. If you're going to pursue small behaviors only, you don't need to concern yourself with motivation. It's not worth the time, effort, or energy to consider getting motivated to do something simple such as walking a block or playing one song on the piano. If you don't feel motivated, you can simply force yourself to do the behavior because it's *that easy*.

In *Elastic Habits*, you will have the same mini habit entry point (and can still use willpower for that), but you also have higher-level goals that will benefit from increased motivation. By stretching our habits laterally and vertically, we're giving ourselves about nine options *per habit*. And each of those nine options has its own motivational profile. How great is that?

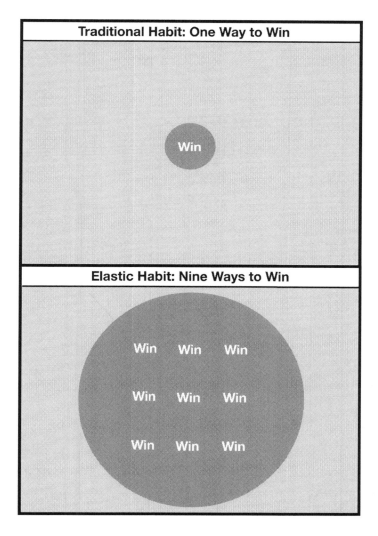

It's exciting, because even if you are motivated to do only *one* of those nine options, you'll still win the day. And don't worry, in the application chapter, I'm going to explain what those nine options are, how to create them, and why it won't be overwhelming to have that many.

Goal sizes are *situationally* good or bad for your motivation. As the Stanford study showed, in certain situations it was helpful to have a small "sub-goal," but in others it hurt more than it helped. This sure seems like a groundbreaking idea. Let's see where it leads.

The Three Motivational Sweet Spots: Attainability, Respectability, Greatness

Imagine a war general saying, "It's *theoretically possible* for us to win the battle and the war, so let's attack right now!" Victory may evade him, as possibility does not guarantee success and he appears to be attacking blindly. Instead, consider this advice, spoken by a legendary war general:

> "First lay plans which will ensure victory, and then lead your army to battle; if you will not begin with stratagem but rely on brute strength alone, victory will no longer be assured."
> ~ Sun Tzu

The proper mindset isn't, "Anything is possible, so I'm going ahead full speed." Instead we must say, "My ultimate goal is possible with the proper strategy, and I will develop it to ensure success." Great strategy comes from superior understanding of the battlefield, so we'll begin with a dissection of how goal motivation works.

Goal Motivation: A Breakdown

If asked why they pursue goals, a person might say, "for the benefits." That's a valid reason to pursue a goal, and benefits do motivate us. But there's one other source of motivation to consider. Let me explain with a couple of whimsical (if mildly disturbing) questions.

1. If you had to either punch a wall or walk on your ceiling right now, which one would you attempt?

Do you have your answer?

I'd bet that you'd punch a wall. Even though punching a wall carries mostly downside, it has the advantage of being imminently more *attainable* than ceiling walking. I think anyone would be impressed if you suddenly started walked on the ceiling, so why not do it? Because while walking on the ceiling is almost certainly more rewarding than punching a wall, it's not attainable because of gravity. You would have to get special equipment to attempt ceiling walking. This highlights *attainability* as a key factor in what motivates us to choose one action over another.

2. If you had to choose between punching a wall and attempting to kiss a rattlesnake (placed in front of you for your convenience), which one would you choose?

I think you'd punch another hole in the wall. In 2017, a Florida man actually did attempt to kiss a rattlesnake. It bit his face and he was airlifted to a hospital. BBC news reported, "It is still not clear why Mr. Reinold tried to kiss the rattlesnake."[1] Indeed, it's difficult to come up with a good reason for kissing an aggressive and highly venomous creature. There's no real value in doing it, only pain, I imagine. I mean, I laughed hard when I read the story, but the snake kisser went to the hospital, so it couldn't have been too funny *for him*.

Trying to kiss a rattlesnake, however, is as easy as leaning in and puckering your lips. It's even less effort than punching a wall! But we will choose wall-punching again, this time for a different reason. Punching a wall takes more effort and thus could be said to be slightly less attainable, but also benefits us more than kissing a rattlesnake (by harming us less). This highlights *action value* as another key factor in what motivates us to take action. Action value is determined by our perceived pain and/or reward from doing it.

Peak attainability and maximum goal value represent two motivational "sweet spots." A motivational sweet spot is a particular level of achievement that contains something specific that we want. If something is extremely attainable and offers even a small benefit, the high attainability can motivate us to action. *We want to always reach our goals.* If something is extremely valuable but difficult to achieve, the sheer value of achieving it can motivate us to action. *We want greater satisfaction and big goal benefits.* By sizing our goals strategically, we can place them right in these sweet spots to encourage action. Then we'll have a buffet of appealing options when it's time to act.

A smart strategy won't require you to conjure up motivation out of thin air. Instead, it will take you to where motivation naturally lies. That's what an elastic habit does. An elastic habit can expand or contract in any direction; unlike single-aim goals, it can reach more than one motivational sweet spot. Let's take a closer look at these motivational sweet spots.

Motivational Sweet Spots
Maximum Attainability (Small Wins): It's desirable to succeed in your pursuits, whatever they are.

Motivated thought: *"I can definitely do that."*

The first thing we consider when thinking about action is usually, "Can I do it? Can I succeed?" It sounds a little bit silly, given that most pursuits are a matter of deciding to act or not. But within the question of "Can it be done?" is the question of "Can I actually get myself to do it?" And in terms of long-term goal pursuit and habit formation, it becomes, "Can I get myself to do it *every day*?" That question is a lot tougher than the one we started with.

It's possible for you to succeed in ways and in magnitudes up to and beyond your wildest dreams. Absolutely, this is a fact. People throughout history have proven it by living fascinating, exciting, and inspiring lives. But possibility can be cruel, too, because if you muse too deeply into what's possible in the future—possibilities for your life are infinite in number—you might miss what's possible in your life *right now*. Actions you can take now are the sure path forward to a better life, and they lead to better future possibilities.

> "It does not do to dwell on dreams and forget to live."
>
> ~ J.K. Rowling, *Harry Potter and the Sorcerer's Stone*

The insatiable lust for theoretical possibility over current reality is a dark and treacherous path into perfectionism and depression. And yet, we live in a world that encourages and celebrates the rejection of reality. People say, "You can do anything if you put your mind to it!"

What if I put my mind to time travel? *Pushes time-travel button after 35 years of work* Hmm ... nothing happened. Now I'm sad and someone owes me 35 years.

Perfectionists are often depressed because their reality

never meets its full potential. *It never will.* You, I, and everyone else in the history of the world have (or had) unreached potential in *every* area of our lives. Yes, we could be better at [everything], but we're not, for many reasons. That's okay, it's the nature of a life of limited time and resources. That gap of possibility will always be there. We can browse possibilities for fun, but let's not get lost in them.

The spectrum of goal attainability goes all the way from automatic win to automatic loss. If you try to clap your hands one time today, you will succeed. It's easily attainable. If you try to swim to the bottom of the Mariana Trench wearing a penguin costume, you will fail (we're talking rattlesnake-kissing levels of failure here). It isn't attainable. Penguin costumes are simply too hard to find. Oh, and the Mariana Trench is 26,850 feet deep.

As your goal moves away from easy attainability, toward improbability, and into impossibility, your motivation to pursue it naturally decreases. The small goal motivational sweet spot lives where the goal is an easily attainable, slightly rewarding step forward. Accomplishing any goal is rewarding because it's a *lot* better than nothing; it either starts a winning streak or keeps one going.

Small goals can withstand practically any deterioration in conditions (whether internal or external). They act as a safety net to catch you on a down day. Anyone who has tried a small step approach like *Mini Habits* knows it's extremely refreshing to win easily *every day*. Your small accomplishments might not look good on paper, but they can change the brain when linked, generate momentum, and are 100% attainable. That's attractive. That's why small goals (when understood and implemented correctly) can naturally motivate us into action. That's one sweet sweet spot.

As we move up the ladder to consider bigger and better things, we need to ask ourselves where the next sweet spot is. Small wins offer the power of ultimate attainability. As we increase the goal's size, at what point will it generate a wholly new benefit? Attainability will decrease as we increase the size of the goal, but will another source of motivation increase to make up for it?

Moderate Attainability Meets Respectability (Medium Wins): A respectable day's work is satisfying and meaningful.

Motivated Thought: *"This is a respectable accomplishment."*

Respectability is the next motivational sweet spot. I'm not saying that a mini habit is unworthy of respect. The consistency, brain-change results, and overall intelligence of the strategy make it a very respectable practice *in the scope of long-term habit development and goal pursuit.* But in the isolated context of a single day, a mini goal may *feel* insignificant.

Since everyone's goals are different, I'll just use myself as a real-life example. If I do a few push-ups, I keep my exercise streak alive. It's great in the scope of my long-term plans, but not a number I'd boast about to my friends the next day. But if I do 30 push-ups, tomorrow I will look back on that amount and feel good about it. Not great. Not ecstatic. Just good. For me, 30 push-ups is decent and that amount of exercise has tangible value in my goal to be healthy and fit.

While medium-sized goals aren't a sure victory as a mini habit is, they are attainable on most days. With the added benefit of being respectable and somewhat substantive, medium goals draw some motivational oomph from both attainability and value. As we move higher up the ladder, attainability will decrease even more. But there's something to make up for it.

Greatness (Large Wins): Who *doesn't* want greatness? Big wins are thrilling. This is the dream.

Motivated thought: *"This is a significant victory and an exciting step forward in my quest for greatness!"*

The next motivational sweet spot can simply be called *greatness*. Whoever you want to be and whatever you want to do is found here. This is because, if you train at something extensively every day, you will master it in time. You will not merely become good at it, but very good or *elite*. Doing something significant on any given day connects you to this dream.

This doesn't apply only to obvious practices like mastering fitness or a new language. You can master having a clean home. You can master idea generation. You can master business correspondence. You can master gardening, playing piano, writing, (speed) reading, mindfulness, and more.

This is the most rewarding, most desirable goal size to reach on any given day, but it's also the least consistently attainable. The people who fail with elastic habits will be the ones who eschew small and medium wins for the idea that "only large wins are acceptable." If you do that, you're merely following every other piece of goal advice that has never worked for you (or at least, it never worked well for me).

This is a special system, because the three distinct goal sizes have their own motivational allure. When you're having a down day, you're going to climb into the arms of attainability. When you're frustrated with mediocrity, you're going to respond by fighting hard for a large and valuable win. When you're somewhere in between, you're going to take the middle ground and be thankful the option is there.

Having three vertical options effectively triples your motivation by opening it up to the full spectrum of attainability to value. But it gets even better. Your motivation will be amplified *even more* than threefold because of phenomenon I call goal anchoring, covered next.

Chapter 5 Closing Thoughts

Motivation has been falling out of favor in habit circles, but that's because rigid goals offer only one form of it. Now that we have three distinct motivators—attainability, respectability, and value—we can find motivation in almost any situation.

Chapter 6
Goal Anchoring for Two-Way Leverage

"Economists point out that the quality of any given option can not be assessed in isolation from its alternatives."

— Barry Schwartz

Ah, slick marketers and salespeople. They ~~are loathsome rapscallions~~ aren't our favorite people, but many of them have an admirable understanding of human psychology under all of that ... grease. One of the oldest, most widespread, and most effective sales techniques ever devised is something called price anchoring. Here's how it works.

I'm going to sell you my car for $240,000. But wait, since you're a friend, I'll take off $50,000. And if you buy in the next 30 minutes, I'll tell you what ... I'll slash the price to only $39,999! That, my friend, is an unbelievable deal. I just knocked over $200,000 off the price of my car. The only thing is, I bought my car new for $32,000. It's not worth $39,999 out of the factory. It only seemed like a bargain for a moment there because I anchored it at $240,000.

Price anchoring happens when someone puts a large price

(or value) on something, even if they don't plan to sell it for that much. The salesperson will play up the product value as expected, and throw out one or more high price points or appraisals of the item's value. Whether you think the price is a rip-off or not matters less than initially associating that price with that item. Through a variety of techniques and explanations, the salesperson will then introduce lower and lower price points, which, in comparison to the original high price(s), look like a great bargain. The key word is *comparison*.

Humans can't help but compare. We compare prices. We compare ourselves to others. We compare Instagram followers and likes on Facebook. Anchoring takes advantage of this relativity in human thought, and *puts the actual price in the most appealing light*. Sales, markdowns, discounts, rebates, coupons, clearances, and limited time offers will never go away. As long as people sell stuff, price anchoring will exist. And if you're in any kind of business, you'd be smart to utilize it.

One of the best examples of anchoring I've seen in a product recently is one that I bought. I never planned to pay almost $200 for a water filter, trust me, but they got me.

While I was neck-deep into trying to figure out which specific contaminants in my water were going to kill me, this company cut through all of the noise with one line: "Drinking Water Filters Optimized for Your City's Water." Sold. On the spot. The price *nearly became irrelevant* at that point. You have dozens of generic water filters, and then you have one company that looks at your city's exact water makeup and customizes your filter for it? Sign me up.

I drink a lot of water and I don't know all the freaky

substances that are in my city's water. Anchored against all of the "dumb" one-size-fits-all water filters, this filter *was custom made for the exact water I drink large quantities of every day.* And to be honest, I don't know how special my customized filter is. It was brilliant anchoring, in any case, and it earned them a sale.

Anchoring Your Goals

A few of my readers have told me that they've felt resistance to doing their mini habits. I've felt it before, too. My knee-jerk response is, "It's *one* push-up. Just do it." But the better response is to ask how and why this could *possibly* happen with such an easy goal.

The benefit of a mini habit is its attainability, or how easy it is to do. The issue is that, like all non-elastic goals and habits, *mini habits aren't anchored to anything.* As the quote at the beginning of this chapter says, "the quality of any given option can not be assessed in isolation from its alternatives."

You can manually compare a mini habit to goals you used to set or could set instead, but that's relatively weak anchoring, because we tend to look at current prices, not hypothetical or past prices. If someone tells you that a baseball card used to be worth $300, but now it's only worth $50 and they'll sell it to you for $35, you're not anchoring to the old $300 value, you're anchoring to the $50, its current perceived value.

When a mini habit becomes your primary strategy, it floats around "as is," anchored to nothing. This is *especially* problematic when your goal is such a screaming-easy win and fantastic value for the effort required! This explains how people can feel resistance to an action they can complete in one minute or less.

We're all used to having goals, and if a mini habit just floats around in your mind as "the current goal/habit strategy you're trying," you're not fully seeing how drastically different it is. It's similar to deciding you're not going to buy anything before you set foot in a store: sometimes people get closed off *to the entire idea* of pursuing goals and habits because they've been burned and disappointed by prior experiences. Here you have something much better, but you may still see it in that same negative light if it isn't anchored to anything for comparison.

Two-Way Leverage

Anchoring is even *more effective* with elastic habits than other applications. Whereas most price anchoring starts with the high price to make the low price more appealing, an elastic habit anchors *both ways, up and down*. That's right. With three goal sizes as options, you gain the power of anchoring in two directions!

First, let's start with how anchoring makes the mini size goal more appealing. I mentioned that the issue with mini habits was that they "floated," and the lack of comparison complicates the perception of how easy these behaviors are to do. Put in another way, the brain might convert "pull one weed in the garden" to a more generic "the annoying thing you have to do today." Both are true, but the latter sure sounds a lot more oppressive, bothersome, and difficult.

With medium and large goals as active options alongside your mini option, you can look at their size and difficulty and see *just how easy* your mini habit is in comparison to them. Instead of looking at a mini habit as your "obligation for the day," you will now see it as it is—a beyond-easy safety net to ensure you never have a losing day. This will *drastically* increase its appeal to you in real time, because from now on, you're deciding *which* goal to do, not *if* you'll do "the one thing you have to do today."

Now for the other direction. Your most ambitious goals will be compared to small and medium-sized goals, making them seem more impressive and feel more substantial when completed. In a typical solo goal setup, regardless of the size of your goal, you're just "doing your job." The fact that it floats alone normalizes it to you. But now, every time you pick the top level, you'll know you're choosing the *hardest option for the greatest reward.* That feels special because *it is freaking special,* and it's made possible by the flexibility of three distinct options creating multiple anchor points for reference.

You can imagine how beneficial this dual leverage is for both keeping you consistent and pushing you to reach higher. When you consider which level you'll do for a behavior on any given day, you will be tempted by the small, easy nature of the mini AND the big, satisfying win of the large, with the middle being a compromise between the two. The pull from both ends of the spectrum keeps it exciting and fresh.

How it Should Feel to Pursue a Goal

Pursuing a goal or habit should feel exhilarating, challenging, explorative, interesting, hopeful, alive, empowering, and even magical. What's more magical than *changing who you are?*

Pursuing a goal or habit should NOT feel restrictive, pointless, overwhelming, burdensome, or lifeless.

If your goal feels more like the latter instead of the former, it means …

- You aren't giving yourself enough freedom.

- You're only doing it for the result.
- You're not playing on your own team.

But when goal pursuit feels right, it means...

- You're giving yourself abundant, empowering freedom, which makes challenges *exciting*.
- You love the process as much or more than the results.
- You're setting yourself up to win, now and later.

The Now and Later Conundrum, Solved by Our Emotions

I know goal pursuit can feel like a lose/lose situation. If you take super-small steps to ensure consistency, it can make you feel like you're not pushing yourself to your full potential. But if you go for outrageously ambitious goals, it can burn you out and keep you from forming lifelong good habits. And the middle ground can feel like a stale compromise that gives you neither the excitement of big goals nor the sureness of small ones.

By having multiple options, *we can counteract whatever negative feeling we're having as we experience it.* Do you feel like you're not doing enough? That's a powerful push to do more and go for a big win. Do you feel like you're getting burnt out and running yourself ragged? That's a great reason to rest a bit and go for the easier win. Do you feel somewhere in the middle? Then push yourself a little, but not too much—a perfect situation for a midrange goal.

Our emotions are fantastic indicators. Let's use them! They can guide us to do the best we can each day. Staying flexible keeps us from feeling as if we're betraying our desires. If you've always felt like you had to fight yourself to do good things, this will be a refreshing and exciting change. There's nothing quite like it.

Often times, I'll find myself start to get frustrated that I'm either doing too much or not enough, and then I'll remember that my habits are elastic and can fully accommodate my desired shift in behavior *that day*. Not only do they accommodate my ups and downs, but they also *reward* my effort, regardless of what I choose to do. After a while, I have no choice but to start thinking, "Hey, I like this!"

I've been more productive than ever before since using the *Elastic Habits* strategy, and that includes my experience with *Mini Habits*. Having an elastic habit feels like a super power because of how effortlessly it pushes you forward. The secret isn't some motivational video that I put together for you to watch every morning at 6 AM, it's *you*. This strategy works with you and for you, however you wish to be worked with! Next we'll cover a few of the infinite possible paths you might take with elastic habits.

Motivational Archetypes

Every person's path to greatness with elastic habits will be different. We're different people with unique motivational styles, habits, and life experiences. Here are just a few of the possible paths to success with this strategy.

> **Terms used:** I'm now going to use the official elastic habit names for the three tiers of success. I call them Mini, Plus, and Elite for small, medium, and large, respectively. Mini is essentially the same as a mini habit, with a bit more lateral flexibility. Plus (medium) comes from the idea that you're doing more than the minimum requirement, even though you don't have to. Elite (large) comes from the idea that if you do this level of activity consistently, you

will become elite in that area.

Here are a few scenarios that could play out with elastic habits. There are an infinite number of possible paths to take, so this is by no means a complete list. You'll also get a preview of how the strategy works (full application directions come later in the book).

The Motivational Snowballer

Jimbo has three elastic habits. He wants to improve his fitness, drink more water, and read more books.

NOTE: For Jimbo's exercise habit, he can walk OR do push-ups OR dance for one song on any given day. He doesn't have to do all three. This is lateral flexibility. The general habit is exercise, and all three of the options below are ways to move forward. Once he picks an activity, he has vertical flexibility and can go for any size win (Mini, Plus, or Elite).

If you look at this first example of exercise in the table below, you'll see nine different success conditions. Isn't that too many options? No, because it's really just *three* options with verticality. Jimbo will choose which exercise he wants to do first, say walking, and then decide how much of it he wants to do depending on the reward he wants and other life factors. Or he'll aim for a certain level of success first, such as the Plus level, and choose an exercise from that tier. There's no wrong way to go about it; it's super-easy (and fun) in practice.

Jimbo's Three Elastic Habits (he picks ONE option for each habit each day. If he walks one block, that satisfies his exercise habit for the day.)

Exercise

Mini	Walk 1 block	2 Push-ups	Dance for 1 song
Plus	Walk 6 blocks	20 Push-ups	Dance for 3 songs
Elite	Walk 20 blocks	50 Push-ups	Dance for 6 songs

Looking at this, doesn't it feel more exciting than a bland, static goal? You know you're going to get a win because of the easy options, but you also have the opportunity for bigger wins!

Some habits don't work well with lateral flexibility or don't need it. There's only one way to drink water (drinking through the nose feels funny), so there's only one option there with three vertical tiers; the same goes for reading.

Drink Water		**Read Books**	
Mini	Drink 1 quart (32 oz.)	Mini	2 pages
Plus	Half gallon (64 oz.)	Plus	15 pages
Elite	Gallon (128 oz.)	Elite	40 pages

Flexible habits are a new concept, so it's important to have an idea of how it might look in practice. I've named Jimbo's journey the "Motivational Snowballer" because he starts off slowly, but gradually builds until it's significant.

Jimbo's Journey (Motivational Snowballer): Jimbo starts out doing the bare minimum (Mini) for all three habits for two weeks straight. He's had a really rough time of it lately and feels like he's at rock bottom, so he's just

66

seeking out some basic wins in the early stages. After two weeks, he looks at his habit tracker and is impressed and encouraged by his consistency.

Jimbo hasn't done a lot on any day yet, but he's done *something* every day and can even feel a small physical difference as a result. I'll never forget realizing an actual difference from doing as little as one push-up a day. When you're at a low point, forward motion in small amounts can feel (and is) meaningful.

On the 17th day, Jimbo gets into a new book called *Elastic Habits 2: Even Stretchier* by Stephen Guise. He reads 43 pages of the book in one day. That's ... an Elite win! That same day, he's feeling good and drinks a half-gallon of water, which earns him a Plus win.

Over the next two weeks, Jimbo earns several more Plus and Elite wins. He's steadily gaining confidence in these key areas and feeling better about himself and his habits every day. He started with just a small snowball, but now it's really rolling and getting bigger. Jimbo's second month continues his momentum—it's absolutely packed with Plus and Elite wins, and he never looks back! Jimbo is a new man.

The Balanced Attacker

Stacy has three elastic habits, because that's what Stephen recommends (it is). Hers are journaling, violin practice, and business. Remember, the numbers she sets below are personal and customized to her.

Journal

Mini	Write 1 sentence	-
Plus	Write 1 paragraph	Write 1 sentence & review one week of entries
Elite	Write 1 page	Write 1 paragraph & review one month of entries

You can get very creative with how you structure each level of victory. Stacy has win options that combine writing and reviewing her journal to encourage both. But since she wants to write in her journal every day, the bare minimum for journal writing is one sentence (her only Mini option).

You may have some lateral options that don't have a Mini level. For example, one of my lateral options for exercise is going to the gym, but that's automatically an Elite win. There is no Mini version of that. If I go to the gym, I always work out for at least 30 minutes, so I don't have a Mini or Plus condition for that particular choice. If your gym workouts vary a lot, you could consider "showing up" at the gym to be a Plus win, and then a certain time or intensity of workout to be Elite.

Violin

Mini	Practice 1 minute	Study music 1 minute	Play 1 song
Plus	Practice 10 minutes	Study music 10 minutes	Play 3 songs
Elite	Practice 30 minutes	Study music 30 minutes	Play 6 songs

Business

Mini	Call 1 lead	Email 1 person (networking)	Write down 2 business ideas
Plus	Call 4 leads	Email 3 people	6 business ideas
Elite	Call 10 leads	Email 7 people	12 business ideas

Stacy's Journey (Balanced Attacker): Stacy, right from the start, has a variety of wins. Looking at her habit tracker, she has accomplished all three sizes of wins from day one. There's no real pattern to see; she just fluctuates between Mini, Plus, and Elite for each habit, depending on the internal and external conditions of her life. She always does her best, and that's good enough!

Stacy continues this mix of wins for three months. After every month, Stacy strategically increases her requirements a bit. She decides that one paragraph of journal writing was too easy for a Plus win, and bumps it up to two paragraphs for the second month. She can do that, because this is *her* system, not a cookie-cutter program that tells her when to tie her shoes. We'll get into Stacy's requirement increase strategy in the "Advanced Tactics" chapter.

The Racehorse

Adelaide is, figuratively speaking, chomping at the bit to start her elastic habits. She owns the *Elastic Habits* book in paperback, ebook, and audiobook and has preordered *Elastic Habits 3: Rubberized Results*. Thanks for the support, Adelaide! Her elastic habits are gratitude, writing, and meditation.

Gratitude

Mini	Write what you're thankful about for 1 minute	Reflect deeply on 1 grateful thought	Thank someone who isn't expecting it
Plus	Thankful writing 3 minutes	Reflect deeply on 3 grateful thoughts	Thank 2 people by person, phone, or email
Elite	Thankful writing 10 minutes	Reflect deeply on grateful thoughts for 15 minutes	Buy or make someone a thoughtful gift

Writing

Mini	Write 50 words	Edit 5 minutes
Plus	Write 500 words	Edit 30 minutes
Elite	Write 1500 words	Edit 2 hours

Mindfulness

Mini	Meditate 1 minute	Yoga with focused breathing for 1 minute
Plus	Meditate 10 minutes	Yoga for 10 minutes
Elite	Meditate 30 minutes	Yoga for 30 minutes

Adelaide's Journey (Racehorse): Adelaide is fired up, and gets at least Plus or Elite in all three habits for the first ten days! She has exceptional momentum, but her motivation and energy dip a couple of weeks into a new pursuit. She starts to feel the pressure of meeting this standard she's seemingly set for herself. For all these reasons, on day 11, she takes a step back and gets the Mini level in all three habits. At first, she's disappointed, then relieved and excited. She realizes that she can take a breather whenever she needs to because the Mini level is so easy, and this supports her go-to-exhaustion ways perfectly.

On day 12, she gets the Mini level in two of three habits. This fires her up a little, because she knows she can do better than that. She goes for another streak of successful Plus and Elite days. Then, she takes a few days off from her torrid pace by focusing on the Mini and Plus level. She continues this sprinting and resting pattern for some time. Despite going a bit too hard for her own good at times, she's still winning every day because she has the flexibility to step back and actively rest at any time.

Everyone's path to success with elastic habits will be unique, and all motivational fluctuations and styles are supported. Personally, I need the Mini level sometimes, but if I see a couple of Mini-heavy days in a row, I do get fired up and often go for at least one Elite win the following day. On multiple occasions, I've even gotten "double Elite," a bonus I created when I did the Elite twice over in one day! I went to the gym for a hard workout and then walked over 15,000 steps later on (both of which are Elite level successes for me). Another day, I wrote 3,000+ words, twice as many as my Elite win condition.

You will also see varying success with each habit. In the first month, I didn't get the Elite level even once with reading. It's not as much of a priority to me as my other habits. If I write for 10 hours or crush it at the gym, I'm okay with not reading a lot. Since reading is something I want to do but struggle to get myself to do, it's been great to have a system that lets me read *something* every day without feeling like a failure.

Chapter 6 Closing Thoughts

Goal anchoring lets you see the true value in small, medium, and large wins. Your path to success with elastic habits will be unique to you, because this isn't an exact recipe you must follow; it's a fun and flexible framework that adapts to your life.

PART FOUR

Smarter Strategy, Superior Results

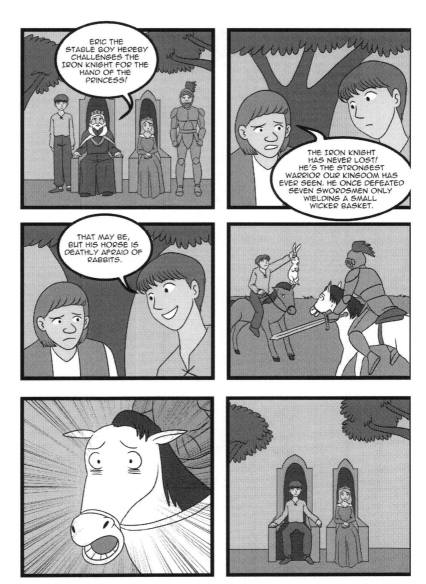

With strong effort, victory is possible.
With strong strategy, victory is inevitable.

Chapter 7
Strategy and System Design

"A vision without a strategy remains an illusion."

— Lee Bolman

Given all that we've covered, we need to discuss system design. You may know all about the power of elastic daily goals (which we have covered in depth), but if you don't strategize a way to make it happen, you've gained nothing. Creating a system to integrate flexible habit pursuit into your life is the next step, and it's more involved. I'm passionate about system design. It was the methodology of *Mini Habits* that made it such a successful book and strategy, not the "small steps help you move forward" aspect of it (which is nothing new).

In this chapter, we will do an overview of the *Elastic Habits* system—what it's like, what makes it work, benefits, what to expect, and so on. This is the strategic backbone that will guide the tactics of your elastic habits. *Elastic Habits* abides by these principles.

1. Intelligent Tracking: Tracking your habits is the most important part of habit formation. It's your accountability and your reward; as a streak lengthens, it deepens your commitment and motivation to continue.

I will show you how to use a standard calendar to track your elastic habits. I've also created a custom elastic habit tracker (for sale at minihabits.com) to make analyzing your progress a joy. It's more effective than other trackers because it divides every month into 15-day halves. (We'll cover February and 31-day months in the application chapter.) I analyzed and tested several time periods. I found one week too short, one month too long, and a full year overwhelming. Roughly two weeks was a perfect time for a checkpoint.

After 15 days, you'll get a score to quantify how you did; you can compare your score to other 15-day periods to see how you're progressing. At the end of the month, you can add your two 15-day periods together to get a monthly score. With the multiple success levels of elastic habits, the scoring component helps motivate greater wins and greater consistency (you get score bonuses for consistency). We'll cover the elastic habit tracker in more detail at the end of the book. It's fun!

2. Simple and Lightweight Execution: There are brilliant systems out there—such as *Getting Things Done* by David Allen—which are phenomenal in design and theory, but fatally flawed in required maintenance for some people. I've tried to implement Allen's GTD system twice in my life, but it was too much for me both times. There are too many components and lots of daily micromanaging involved. I'm still a big fan of the book and the ideas in it, such as his famous two-minute rule (if it takes two minutes or less, do it without thinking).

I believe in minimizing the time and number of actions required to keep a habit system going. I'll put it this way: Once the *Elastic Habits* system is (quickly and easily) set up, every interaction you have with it will be short, fun, and rewarding (not tedious or time-intensive). To maintain the system, it will literally take you less than 20 seconds per day. If you score yourself every 15 days as recommended, that takes about two minutes of your time every two weeks. That's easy and sustainable for life, and the rewards are immense.

3. Life-Aware Methodology: A smart system considers solutions for all possible situations. This one is based in the reality of a modern, busy, and stressful life, not idealist fantasy. You'll find solutions for vacations, missed days, and so on. And flexibility being the core feature of the system means it is naturally 10 times more "life-aware" than other static goal methods.

4. Goal and Intention Tangibility: Habit formation is typically lacking in one area—the senses. Elastic habits feature real-world environment integration. In other words, your daily goals and habits can "exist" in the real world in the form of habit posters. You can even interact with them, as I'll discuss in the product section at the back of the book.

5. Automatic Problem Solving: There are a lot of problems we encounter when pursuing goals and habits; most of them are internal. We make excuses, we want perfect action (and do nothing as a result), we get sick of following the same boring goals that we set months ago, we procrastinate and postpone our dreams, we lose motivation, and so on. Many books and systems attempt to guide you through overcoming these issues individually. This can help, but there's something even better.

This system and methodology are designed to *automatically* overcome these issues. For example, excuses are destroyed by the Mini level option (it's too easy for excuses). Perfectionists can find satisfaction in having every day in their tracker filled. The motivational sweet spots can motivate you in *multiple* ways. And finally, the system stays fresh and adapts with you, keeping your interest.

Good design facilitates the fixing of problems; great design solves problems *before* they happen. You won't be tasked with micromanaging the internal roadblocks that often emerge from stale, rigid, brittle goals. You'll find that your most common roadblocks disappear when you use this system as intended.

6. Lateral Flexibility: The original *Mini Habits* had some lateral flexibility in what I called hybrid mini habits. Elastic habits are more expansive, encouraging several lateral options per habit (if desired or useful). Examples:

- Guitar: study music theory, practice chords, practice songs
- Exercise: weightlifting, cardio (do HIIT!), stretching/yoga, sports, active rest days (walk, swim, etc.)
- Writing: write content, edit content, research, market your work
- Cleaning: clean and organize an area or whole room, do one type of cleaning (dust, vacuum, scrub, etc.), get rid of unwanted items (declutter), pick things up off the floor.

In addition to those listed, the timed option works for just about any habit (e.g., clean for one minute). Here are a couple of examples of why flexible options make the difference between daily success and awkward, forced breaks (as is the case in other strategies).

When you start playing guitar, the soft skin of your fingertips can hurt and even bleed from pressing on the strings. You need to give your fingers some time to toughen up, and, if they're bleeding, you will be forced to rest them. With lateral flexibility, you can still pursue guitar every day by studying music theory as your fingers recover.

There are practically unlimited ways to exercise. One issue I (and others) have found when trying to form an exercise habit is that identical daily repetition isn't usually suitable for training. If you do high-intensity interval training or weight training or any other higher-intensity work, you are going to need recovery days. Even workout warriors such as Dwayne Johnson rest weekly.

With elastic habits, you can make your exercise habit a daily affair because of lateral flexibility. If it's a rest day, you can go for a walk or a light swim to meet your requirement. Whatever your condition or injury situation, an elastic habit always allows you to do *something*. Better yet, as you'll see in the next principle, it even enables you to get **Elite** wins on your rest days. Because lateral flexibility is built into the strategy, there's no guilt or second-guessing when surprises interfere with your plans. You can pivot your activity on any day and keep your winning streak alive.

Here's how great this is. I live in Orlando next to the major theme parks. My three elastic habits are reading, writing, and exercise. If I want to spend the entire day in the theme park, I can meet all of my daily goals (which are usually done at home or the gym) *at the theme park*.

- **Exercise:** Walking counts for me. If I wanted to, I could walk every single day to meet my exercise goal (walking is fantastic, fundamental, and functional exercise). My levels of success are 5, 10, or 17 thousand steps for Mini, Plus, and Elite, respectively. A full day at the theme park is a lot of walking, and I'm rewarded for being active. Modern smartphones can count your steps automatically. I use Google Fit, the built-in step counter for Android. Apple iPhones also track steps through the Health app. You can download a number of other pedometer apps for different graphics and features as well.

- **Writing:** I can write on my phone in a dedicated phone app (I use Google Keep) to meet my requirement anywhere. Later, I can transfer it to my computer.
- **Reading:** I read books on my phone, and standing in line for a ride is a great opportunity to do that!

I never feel trapped, only empowered and free. Not all habits will be doable outside of the home, but many can be adapted in some way. I hope that you'll embrace the spirit of this strategy to find more ways to win in areas that matter to you.

Elastic habits will open your eyes to new opportunities in more places and situations. With a flexible strategy, you'll find ways to get that daily win when circumstances are less than ideal. If I can't meet any of my exercise options for some reason (full body cast?), I will try to create a temporary new option. Bargaining is not merely allowed with elastic habits, it's encouraged. With a normal goal, an adaptation like this feels like you've failed (and by the structure of an all-or-nothing rigid goal, you have). See the difference? Find success every day, in one of many ways. Adapt and conquer!

7. Vertical Flexibility: Vertical flexibility is just as important as lateral flexibility. An elastic habit can expand and contract, from spectacular highs to moderate middles to very easy lows.

As discussed in chapter 6, vertical flexibility creates valuable anchor points for reference. Anchor points make small goals seem smaller (easier) and large goals seem larger (more rewarding). I call it two-way leverage because you can reference the large option to make the small option seem easier, and reference the small option to make the large option more impressive.

It's important that vertical flexibility is defined specifically. For example, saying "I'll run" covers the spectrum of all possible distances and offers unlimited vertical flexibility, but gives you no incentive or reason to run any particular distance. Saying that you'll run one mile is better. Saying that you'll run either a quarter of a mile, one mile, or three miles every day is best.

Adding vertical flexibility to your goals is like adding fresh herbs and spices to a bland dish. It makes the whole experience more exciting, day after day. Surprises are plentiful!

With vertical flexibility, you always have a way to rest or push your limits. You always have a way to prioritize one behavior if the situation calls for it.

8. Alive Goals: What happens when you set a typical goal? It doesn't change. It doesn't move. It freezes in that moment. It basically dies. It's boring and feels like work soon after it's created.

You decide to practice piano an hour per day and that's it. You hope to meet that standard each day, and the best-case scenario is that you meet it most of the time. An elastic habit is more fun than that!

On any day with an elastic habit, you may surprise yourself with a "double Elite" or "Elite+" win. Again, that's where you meet the Elite level (the highest) and then *meet it again on the same day.* It's a huge win, and it feels good to give yourself full credit for it (it includes a point bonus if you keep score).

Over time, you can strategically move your targets up, down, and sideways. You might even swap out your lateral options just to keep it fresh. For example, if you've primarily been doing yoga, you can switch to plyometrics for a bit. Having a system like this one makes these shifts seamless.

9. Naturally Rewarding Experiences: External rewards are a staple of habit formation systems, but a well-designed system will need no (or minimal) external rewards to reinforce the behavior. That's because there are so many built-in rewards in habit pursuit.

1. Any winning, non-zero day is encouraging.
2. Every outsized win feels exhilarating.
3. Seeing yourself change for real is thrilling.
4. Winning streaks over days, weeks, and months are empowering.
5. Each behavior has unique rewards (endorphins from exercise, knowledge from reading, calmness from meditation, etc.).

Reaching your most exciting goals and forming life-changing habits is more rewarding than any extrinsic reward could ever hope to be. Transforming your brain and behavior for the better is one of the greatest feelings in the world. The issue is, of course, that it's not usually tangible until you've arrived. I've created tools to change that. You won't merely see, but also *feel and express* your success with elastic habits (more on this in the products section). Now, let's discuss strategy and tactics.

Goals Inform Strategy, Strategy Informs Tactics

The following quote by Sun Tzu from chapter 4 is extremely important. It highlights the fact that strategy is the true engine of victory.

> "All men can see the tactics whereby I conquer, but what none can see is the strategy out of which victory is evolved. **Do not repeat the tactics which have gained you one victory, but let your methods be regulated by the infinite variety of circumstances.**"

If there's a single statement that defines this book, it's this one, notably the bolded part. *Elastic Habits* is a strategy, which is why your tactics (what you do and how much of it you do) will change daily. This is so important to point out because so many people solely focus on tactics.

You can watch someone succeed, but just because you've seen their tactics does not mean that you can replicate their success. As Tzu implies, it's more difficult to know and understand the strategic thinking that drives those tactics. Here's a famous example of why you can't trust tactics alone.

The Game of the Century

In what's now called "The Game of the Century," a 13-year-old chess prodigy named Bobby Fischer played against 26-year-old Robert Byrne. This game became famous because Byrne's bishop attacked Fischer's queen, the most powerful and second most valuable piece in chess. Instead of moving and protecting his queen as most players would do, Fischer moved his bishop. Byrne made the obvious move next—he took Fischer's queen. At this point, viewers and expert commentators thought Fischer had lost the game. It looked like a bizarre tactical mistake.

Immediately after taking Fischer's queen, however, Byrne proceeded to get shellacked by Fischer's knight and bishop. He put Byrne in check repeatedly, taking away Byrne's ability to maneuver and removing many of Byrne's key pieces in the process. Fischer initially seemed crazy (as I did when I used to do one push-up per day), because giving up your queen, generally speaking, *is crazy*. But Fischer's brilliance in that game (and his chess career as a whole) came from his ability to strategize on a deeper level than his opponents. Ultimately, he gave up his queen in exchange for *several pieces* that were less valuable individually but more valuable collectively. Fischer won the game easily. It was a good trade after all.

Notice that Fischer's key tactic—sacrificing his queen—was bound to the context of that specific game. All tactics are bound by context, which is why those who copy tactics will have wildly different results. They all have different contexts. For real results and true success, *you must always use strategy to inform your tactics*. Intelligent tactics aren't copied or born out of thin air; they're crafted directly from strategy. If you want to mimic someone, look beyond their tactics (what they do) and into their strategy (*why they do what they do in those specific contexts*).

The typical person has a few general goals nailed down. They know they want to get healthier, garden more, improve their violin skills, and read more books (or something). But then they'll settle for simplistic tactics without strategy.

"Lose 50 pounds" is not a strategy, it's a slightly more specific (but still general) iteration of "lose weight." If the person declares something like that as their strategy, their actual strategy is, "Do stuff that results in weight loss." Yikes. What's stuff? *How* is that done? What if something goes wrong? It'd be like a war general saying, "Defeat the enemy by gittin' 'em real good." General Tzu wouldn't approve.

Actual strategies involve analyzing your strengths and weaknesses, looking at potential obstacles and opportunities (your environment), and devising a plan that gives you the greatest chance of success within common *and* uncommon contexts. A great strategy will consistently put you in advantageous situations and leverage your effort. A 30-day challenge is not good strategy; it's a pop-culture trend only slightly better than the "git 'em good" strategy.

Most strategies out there are so bad that they only work when you're at your best. So, what is a good strategy for setting and achieving goals and forming habits? Perhaps Sun Tzu, arguably the greatest war strategist in history, can offer us some wisdom.

Sun Tzu's Five Essentials to Victory

You probably have noticed by now that Sun Tzu is one of my favorite historical figures. His *The Art of War* is a masterpiece of strategy that doesn't only apply to war. War is an apt metaphor for many aspects of life. We battle against ourselves to do the right things. We battle against circumstances that stand in our way. We battle against limitations of time, energy, and resources. You could say that every day is a battle of our ideal life against the various forces—internal and external—that keep us from it.

There is plenty of metaphorical war to be found in personal development, and thus plenty of valuable concepts to be learned from a master strategist like Tzu. In *The Art of War*, Tzu gives five essentials for victory. I have adapted these essentials to daily battles in the war to build better habits and lives. The ever-changing tactics of someone following *Elastic Habits* looks different from most others you'll see because they are *deeply strategic*, and founded upon proven concepts that have been used for millennia.

Sun Tzu says, "There are five essentials for victory:

1. He will win who knows when to fight and when not to fight.
2. He will win who knows how to handle both superior and inferior forces.
3. He will win whose army is animated by the same spirit throughout all its ranks.
4. He will win who, prepared himself, waits to take the enemy unprepared.
5. He will win who has military capacity and is not interfered with by the sovereign."[1]

Let's cover these, one by one.

1. He will win who knows when to fight and when not to fight.

In war, timing is crucial. The difference between attacking when you have the advantage and when you do not is often the difference between victory and defeat.

If you set a flat, rigid goal, you cannot follow this strategy in your life. Rigid goals require you to fight the same battle the same way every day. On disadvantaged days, you'll lose the battle, and every lost battle makes losing the war more likely. On advantaged days, you might not fight aggressively enough. Any strategic prowess you may have is strangled because a rigid goal is a single tactic; with one tactic, there is little strategic maneuvering.

An elastic habit provides the flexibility necessary to heed Tzu's wisdom here. If it's not the right day to fight hard, you can simply meet the easy Mini requirement (a tactical shift to stay in the fight) and perhaps prepare for a later strike.

When the time does come to fight, you have the tools and incentives to win big (a tactical shift for greater progress). Fighting when you're prepared produces the best results and the most satisfaction. Specifically, that difference is in your preparedness to win. When you attempt an Elite win, you will almost always get it. Why? Because it's done on your terms, and you can do all you need to ensure victory.

2. He will win who knows how to handle both superior and inferior forces.

By this, Tzu meant that you need to know how to handle situations in which your army is superior or inferior to the enemy's army. The situations call for drastically different (opposite) strategies and tactics.

The Art of War commentator Chang You says, "By applying the art of war, it is possible with a lesser force to defeat a greater, and vice versa. The secret lies in an eye for locality, and in not letting the right moment slip. Thus Wu Tzu says: "With a superior force, make for easy ground; with an inferior one, make for difficult ground."[2]

In war, the idea here is to choose the proper terrain based on the current strength of your army relative to your opponent's army.

This is a brilliant metaphor for the lateral flexibility of elastic habits. My fitness elastic habit includes both intense exercise and "active rest" exercise. It can be completed at the gym or at home. If I feel strong, I can go to the gym and exercise hard. But the next day, I might need to recover my strength, so I can take an active rest day and walk around my local lake. Elastic habits allow you to alter *the application, terrain, and intensity* of your habit, depending on your current situation. You will choose your terrain based on how your current strength compares to the challenges and obstacles of the day.

3. He will win whose army is animated by the same spirit throughout all its ranks.

This is, in a word, unity. For an army to succeed, all units need to be on the same team, in the same spirit. Unity strengthens bonds, communication, vigor, and loyalty, top to bottom, from officers to line soldiers.

An elastic habit also needs and benefits from unity between the three ranks of Mini, Plus, and Elite. Some people may use this system and immediately gravitate towards the Elite only, and devalue the other two. What happens to an army when the lowly foot soldiers are treated poorly and taken for granted? In a key moment, they may turn away instead of fight, as they have been given no reason to be loyal to their superiors. Just as every part of an army unites to make the whole stronger, each level of success you can attain with an elastic habit contributes to your ability to do more of the things that matter to you (and make them into habits).

I recommend color-coded stickers for tracking your elastic habits (more on this in the application chapter) because they are uniform in size and shape. (It's no coincidence that armies wear uniforms.) They all look the same except for the color nuance to indicate their rank, just as small pins, badges, stripes, or color differences denote rank in armies. This shows that all levels are equally important and viable contributors for the most critical objective: filling that space and getting the win each day. The Elite level is not always better than the Plus level, because the Plus level will work best for you in certain situations.

4. He will win who, prepared himself, waits to take the enemy unprepared.

If you are more prepared for battle than your enemy, it's likely a good time to strike. But Tzu says the key word of "wait" here. He doesn't say to strike immediately when *you're prepared*, but to also wait until *the enemy is unprepared* for your attack to maximize your advantage.

In the war of behavior change, I see this as the long game, with our own brains as the "enemy preventing positive change." Your brain isn't a true enemy to you, but an ally. It will, however, act as an enemy and stop you if you overwhelm it with challenging new behaviors.

The subconscious mind resists all changes at first. It's perfectly content to do what it has always done. Thus, it is always prepared to stop any aggressive attempt you make to change for the better. Habit formation strategies like this one change the brain at a pace it will allow.

In your journey to form better behavioral patterns, it may be tempting to quickly and dramatically increase all of your targets to high levels. But if you haven't formed the neural pathways to support those behaviors, they will be overtaken by your previous behavioral preferences. Be patient as you pursue change. It can't happen quickly, so it's best to embrace that.

As you move forward with elastic habits, you will increasingly prepare yourself for mastery in these areas while, at the same time, your brain will begin changing to accept them. Thus, you will become more prepared to reach the next level as your brain becomes less prepared to stop you from doing it. It happens simultaneously.

I know you are consciously prepared to transform your life right now, but you must wait for your subconscious brain and habits to change before you *attack* your goals like a berserker. Be patient and accept the victories you can get right now. If you're consistent, you will prevail in the long game.

5. He will win who has military capacity and is not interfered with by the sovereign.

Sun Tzu saved the best for last. Wang Tzu said in regards to this, "It is the sovereign's function to give broad instructions, but to decide on battle it is the function of the general."[3]

For a general to succeed in military operations, he needs the freedom to make decisions based on real-time conditions. This book is giving you the broad instructions, the tools, and the knowhow to succeed in the war of behavior change. The whole idea of elastic habits is to give you the daily freedom you need to win battles every day so that you can ultimately win the war. I'm one author speaking to readers with very different lives, and no reader will ever live the same two days, let alone the same day as another reader. You are the general who will decide each day, laterally and vertically, what type and size of victory you will achieve for each habit.

The sovereign could be seen as the typical goal or program that tells you exactly what to do at all times. When you follow a strict program like that, you have no input and can't do your job as the general, which is to look at the battlefield of your life and adjust your strategy. With elastic habits you can, and you're going to love the difference.

Would Sun Tzu Approve of Elastic Habits?

Looking broadly at Sun Tzu's essentials to victory, they all involve having the freedom to stay flexible and take strategic actions based on conditions of each army, the terrain, and factors like preparedness. If he were to create a goal or habit formation strategy, I believe it would look a lot like *Elastic Habits*. I will never know for sure, since Tzu died in 496 BC, just a few years before I was born, but the principles sure do fit.

No other strategy gives us such flexibility and freedom to maneuver every single day. No other strategy gives us the autonomy to craft a unique path to victory based on the reality of our lives. No other strategy gives us a better chance to win the war of behavior change.

Chapter 7 Closing Thoughts

Some days are about not losing. Others are about winning. This system gives you the flexibility for both options and everything in between. There's no situation in which you will feel unprepared. Next, we'll look at the risks and ramifications of adding flexibility and choice to life.

Chapter 8
The Ramifications of Choice

"There's no question that some choice is better than none. But it doesn't follow from that that more choice is better than some choice."

— Barry Schwartz

There is great value in both stability and flexibility, but the greatest value comes from combining them. A totally rigid body can't move because it has no flexion. A totally flexible body can't move itself because it has no stable structure to flex *with or against*. At the extremes, you have either an iron bar or a puddle on the floor. In the middle, you have much of the animal life we see in the world—dynamic and powerful creatures made by combining stability and flexibility. Stability gives structure and control. Flexibility gives options and maneuverability. We need both!

The shoulder joint is our least stable joint, which is how it moves so dynamically! But the difference between low stability (healthy) and *zero* stability (dislocation) in the shoulder joint is the difference between a baseball pitcher throwing a 99 mph fastball and not being able to move his arm at all.

Hips are our most stable joint, and consequently require

relatively little energy to support us while standing. Try walking around on your hands for a few minutes, and your shoulder joint will take on the role of your hips in supporting your body. I'm sure you'll feel the difference in energy expenditure!

Elastic Habits: The "Super Joint"

If *Elastic Habits* had no structure, it would be like saying, "Do whatever you want and however much of it you want at any time! Whatever and whenever! Total flexibility, Broseph!"

It's easy to see how useless that is because *that's what people without plans for their life already do*. But we're trying to make our goal and habit pursuit dynamically powerful, like the shoulder, with a strong enough structure to use and protect that power.

An elastic habit may be the most flexible habit you've ever seen, but it has some stability, too. It's like a "super joint," because it has the powerful mobility of the shoulder joint and the low-energy consumption and stability of the hip joint.

The Energy Cost of Stability

The hip's stability allows us to stand without using significant muscle contraction, saving us energy. The question is, what is the equivalent of muscle contraction in goal and habit pursuit? What is it that drains our energy?

We've covered the cost of having no stability—that's the blob on the floor or the aimless person. But adding stability to a goal or habit plan isn't free: it carries an energy cost. Unlike the human body, in goal systems, *it's rigidity that costs us energy*. Why? Rigidity (or stability) means that *you* must adapt to your goal, requiring more effort from you for success. Flexibility means that *your goal* adapts to you, requiring less effort from you for success.

A simple example: What can happen with a person who decides to run one mile every day (rigid goal) compared to a person who has an exercise elastic habit (flexible goal within a stable structure)?

Day 1: Dani is busy, tired, and has a deadline to meet.

- A standard goal forces her to run one mile.
- An elastic habit allows for a quick Mini win. She dances to one song.

Day 2: Dani has the time, motivation, and energy to run.

- A standard goal forces her to run one mile again.
- An elastic habit can expand into a two mile run. She runs two miles!

In this example, Dani ran the same amount with each strategy—two miles in two days. But notice how differently each situation is building.

The elastic habit gave Dani freedom to do less on the first day and more on the second day, which matched the flow of her life. It was *precisely* what she needed to feel encouraged, empowered, and excited for more. The rigid habit was comparatively stubborn, forcing Dani to run the same amount on a busy day as she did on a wide open day.

With the standard goal, Dani is now in danger of becoming *resentful* of her schedule and/or her goals, because she values both, but they interfere with each other. And she's right to feel that way, because her goal is rigid and asks too much of her on some days and not enough of her on other days. It will likely fail.

As you can see, rigid goals take a lot of energy and brute force to maintain. Flexible goals take much less energy because they *always* fit your life. Let's keep in mind that Dani wants to run and get in shape. The elastic habit amplifies that desire by working with her and encouraging her every day, while the standard goal abuses her desire and suffocates it with a rigid rule.

Thus, we need to be very careful and precise with structure, because excess structure (rigidity) can threaten our sense of power, control, and freedom.

The Four Pillars of Elastic Habits (Structure)

The following four items are the structural pieces of *Elastic Habits*. I've harped on about flexibility in the book to this point, so please notice how *inflexible* these are, while still allowing the flexible aspects of the system to shine.

The First Pillar: Elastic habits are to be done *every day*. This is a hard and unyielding key to success with this system. How and when you do them each day is flexible, but they must be done! In most systems, *every day* sounds intimidating. But it's not so intimidating once you realize you can complete the Mini level in less than a minute. You can do it right before jumping into bed if you forgot to do it earlier. Intimidation gone. Streak maintained.

The Second Pillar: Elastic habits have a *limited number* of lateral and vertical success points. I found that three levels of vertical success is *dramatically* better than four. Just like with human joints, there's a point where increased flexibility does more harm than good. This isn't an unlimited spectrum of possible win conditions; it's turning the typical *single* success point into about *nine* success points, as shown in this graphic from earlier in the book.

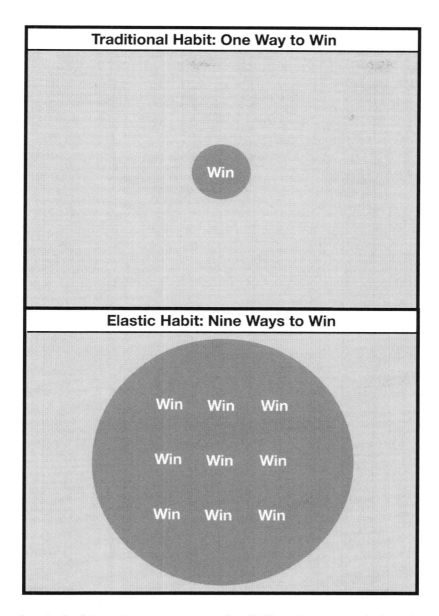

Elastic habits give you *more* flexibility than usual, but it's not even close to a puddle on the floor. It's good to have more than one win condition. But it's important to limit them too (lateral options x vertical tiers = 3x3 = 9 win conditions). Structure and flexibility work together.

The Third Pillar: Elastic habits need to be tracked. You can't just do this in your head and expect to change. Tracking is as simple as placing three stickers on paper every day (if you use the official elastic habit tracker). The stickers are color coded to represent your earned tier of success. Tracking your habits every day does several things to make this work.

Tracking both validates your success and excites you for the higher tier levels. Checking off the *same habit every day* is mildly satisfying, but it gets boring. Back when I did only mini habits, I started off tracking with exclamation points, motivational phrases, and high general enthusiasm. A month later, it was just check marks. That's fine, but it shows that, even while succeeding, my excitement waned.

Having the option to get a massive, Elite win and claim that victory by marking it is super exciting (months into it, I can confirm this does not get old!). We'll cover the tracking system in more detail in the last chapter of the book. While tracking is a must, tracking elastic habits is very easy and far more rewarding than other habit tracking, so it's more a pleasure than a burden.

The Fourth Pillar: Have no more than three elastic habits at one time. If you want maximum success with this system, you'll get it by focusing your efforts on important habits. As I said in *Mini Habits*, as you increase your number of actively pursued habits, you divide your energy and focus among them. If you have too many habits, your energy and focus will become too diluted to be effective.

It's worthwhile to pursue multiple habits, because, let's

face it, nobody wants to do one habit at a time. There are probably 89 things you want to pursue right now! But start with the most impactful ones, such as exercise, skill-building, meditation, reading, writing, business, relationships, and so on. Once you start reaping the benefits of these most important habits, I promise you won't regret focusing on them.

Later we will cover options for contextual elastic *actions*, but for the core habit-building system, the one that will transform your daily life, keep it to three elastic habits maximum for the best results.

Those four things are the only rigid and stabilizing components of *Elastic Habits*. Everything else will flex and bend around your life and your preferences.

1. Do your elastic habits daily.
2. Limit your lateral and vertical flexibility to three options each.
3. Track your success.
4. Have no more than three elastic habits at a time (an exception for a non-habit plan will be discussed later).

Dealing with the Paradox of Choice and Decision Fatigue

There's only one apparent weakness in this strategy as a whole—you must decide what to achieve each day. Creating multiple targets introduces extra choices into your life, something we usually don't want or need. It brings up two potential issues called *choice paralysis* and *decision fatigue*. First, let's discuss choice paralysis.

Choice Paralysis: A Consequence of Trivial Excess

Psychologist Barry Schwartz has made the point that excessive choices costs us happiness. In his popular TED Talk, Schwartz mentions his local grocery store has 175+ different salad dressings.[1]

> "With a lot of salad dressings to choose from, if you buy one and it's not perfect—and what salad dressing is?—it's easy to imagine that you could have made a different choice that would have been better. And what happens is, this imagined alternative induces you to regret the decision you made and this regret subtracts from the satisfaction you get out of the decision you made, even if it was a good decision."

This phenomenon, and anticipating the regret to come, causes choice paralysis. With too many options, it's nearly impossible to pick "the best one." We know this, and it eats away at our souls. I'm not proud to share this, but one night, I spent more than 20 minutes looking at *rice* in the grocery store, and that's a freaking commodity! Even as a commodity, there are many types of rice—basmati, jasmine, white, brown, long grain, short grain, and several different brands carry each variety!

> "I MUST PICK THE BEST RICE AT THE IDEAL INTERSECTION OF QUALITY, TASTE, HEALTH, VALUE, AND PRICE! Oh, they have quinoa, too?"
> ~ My thoughts in a grocery store

The modern world has inundated us with choice, but the problem isn't choice itself. After all, being able to choose is the very mark of *freedom*. Slavery is defined as having no choice or self-governance. Therefore, freedom and choice are inseparable, and, given the absolute importance of freedom, choice itself can't be the issue. So what is? There are two sub-issues with choice in the modern world— triviality and lack of restraint.

Trivial choices aren't worth making. When you go to buy ketchup and see 20 bottles that are basically the same thing with minor differences in price, quality, ingredients, and packaging, you aren't making a life-altering choice. The companies that market these products do a very good job of making it *feel* like you are, but it's a trivial decision. Even if you want to buy ketchup with better or organic ingredients, *there are multiple choices within that category.* Trivial choices like these can frustrate us because we know they usually aren't worth the time and energy it takes to make them.

Unrestrained choices overwhelm the mind. With all choices, *especially trivial ones,* it's best to reduce the number of options as quickly and efficiently as possible. This takes the pressure off identifying the best ones (with fewer choices, the odds of choosing the best one go up and our odds of regret and overthinking go down). Since the grocery store isn't going to help us out, we generally pre- filter our choices to prevent ourselves from going insane.

Here's an example of a good filter that I use often: "The Dirty Dozen" and "Clean Fifteen" by the Environmental Working Group.[2] The Dirty Dozen lists the most pesticide- laden conventionally grown fruits and vegetables, and the Clean Fifteen tells you what conventional produce has little or no pesticide residue. Organic food is expensive, so this filter helps me save money and feel good about my choices. If it's avocados or onions, I buy conventional because they are part of the "Clean Fifteen." If it's strawberries or spinach, I buy organic because they test high for pesticide residue. That filter makes the decision easy for me.

As for everything else, here's the secret to life (or one of them). It's rarely about choosing the very best one. It's about choosing a good or very good one and being happy with it. I'm an author now and love it, but I know I may have been happier as a professional shark wrestler. At the very least, I'd be tan and have a shark-tooth necklace and a peg leg. Joking aside, I can think of a couple other careers I might enjoy more than this one, but *I love this one*. I have no reason to fret, regret, or complain. There's always something better out there, but good doesn't become bad in the presence of great.

Much of the unhappiness and regret Schwartz refers to is the result of excessive choices heightening our awareness of the fact that we probably won't pick the best one. Just keep in mind, even if you pick the worst salad dressing option, *if you like it, you still made a good decision!*

Decision Fatigue
Scientific studies have shown that making decisions wears us down to a certain extent. This makes sense, since we use brain power to make choices. To consider the decision fatigue cost of your daily elastic habits, we need to put it in context.

It's important not to put this system in a vacuum, because it's a superior *replacement* for whatever habit system you're currently using. Every goal or habit formation system has an "energy cost" to manage and execute it. The key question is whether or not the system helps you enough to justify its energy cost.

In every other system I've ever seen, the objective is stationary and unchanging, and that has the significant cost of *rarely meshing with your day-to-day reality*. It takes an enormous amount of mental energy to do something that you know doesn't fit today's agenda or at least not at its current capacity. Even with the easy *Mini Habits* strategy, on days that you feel you can achieve a lot, it can be frustrating to see your goal of "one push-up" just because it's so far from your reality in that moment.

When your goal doesn't fit your day, it's exhausting because there isn't a single good response! If your rigid goal doesn't work with your situation, here are your options. They're not good.

1. You can change your goal, which challenges the entire idea of having a static goal in the first place. If you can go about changing your one goal whenever you want, then your initial static goal had no meaning and no reason to be static. That's awkward.

2. You can adapt yourself and your schedule to the goal and do it anyway. You'll have to cancel plans and you'll resent the goal (eventually) for not being at all adaptable. Resentment of static goals builds over time because they demand the same thing from you regardless of your situation. Every time you force action that doesn't make sense for your situation, you'll wonder if your goal is right for you. If a change of schedule springs up, you will be frustrated that your goal(s) can't accommodate it well.

3. You can skip a day. If your goal is meant to be ironclad (and it should be if you want results), skipping it is a clear failure and the prerequisite to quitting. Even if your goal is designed to have built-in, flexible skip days, having only one measure of victory creates an all-or-nothing situation, leaves progress on the table, kills habit formation, and makes losing streaks likely if not inevitable.

There's no need to dig too deeply into those ramifications. They're only there to show you how quickly complicated and *exhausting* a static goal can get when you try to fit it into your dynamic life. We tend to design our strategies with the perfect day in mind, which means we're screwed when the "perfect storm" hits on Monday, Thursday, and Friday. But a perfect storm isn't necessary, because normal life is more than enough to disrupt our plans (I sprained my ankle the day I wrote this).

When you're forced to improvise with a static goal that is designed for predictability, disaster is inevitable. The whole framework falls apart, like a brittle material that reaches its elastic limit (e.g., glass shattering). There's no easy way to make static goals work well, which is why they live and die like flies. Like most weak-but-unyielding things, they're not built to survive for very long in your dynamic life, in this dynamic world.

Every decision carries an energy cost. The cost is determined by how difficult the decision is. When your goal is rigid, the assumed decision to do the behavior can wind up being more difficult than the decision you make with a flexible goal.

How Elastic Habits Overcome Choice Paralysis and Decision Fatigue
Choice paralysis is caused by triviality and unrestrained choices.

Elastic habit choices are not trivial. On a difficult day, your ability to choose an easier option keeps your streak alive and keeps you engaged. On a high-motivation day, the option to get the enticing big win helps you achieve more than you usually would. *Elastic habits introduce choice into an area that desperately needs it.* We don't need 47 types of ketchup that are all the same, but we do need multiple types of goals to maximize every unique day.

As for choices, I initially designed a habit poster with four levels of vertical success (Mini, Plus, Mega, and Elite). I had the poster designed, took it to a printer, and finally held it in person. As soon as I thought about picking one of the four levels, it felt like I was trying to buy rice again. How much better was Mega than Plus? Or Elite than Mega? How much is each one worth compared to the effort needed to reach it? How will I know?

When I cut it down to three sizes (Mini, Plus, Elite), the difference was immediate and immense. We're all familiar with small, medium, and large sizes, and so we can quickly parse those options and what they mean in relation to each other. That's the difference between a life-changing strategy and a broken one. Limiting choice is that important.

I'm aware of choice paralysis and carefully designed this strategy with it in mind. You won't have a problem with it! The same goes for decision fatigue.

An elastic habit has complete lateral and vertical flexibility, letting you select the one activity and intensity that fits your situation today, *right now*. Importantly, these options are *limited* and parked at motivational sweet spots (as described in chapter 5). Having limited options with clear decision criteria effectively mitigates decision fatigue, especially when compared to standard, inflexible goals.

It's like having a neatly organized toolbox with everything you could possibly need to succeed. When you're working on a house project, it's not a burden to have a hammer, a wrench, *and* a screwdriver—you just select the one you need when you need it. Elastic habits are the same way.

I have about 15 shirts and only one pair of jeans so that I don't have to think much about what to wear. I have only one type of socks so that I can grab any two and go. The point is, I ruthlessly remove decisions from my life, but the elastic habit decisions I make every day are fun and intuitive to make! Elastic habits are a beacon of flexibility and freedom in a dark world full of rigid and brittle goals.

While choice paralysis and decision fatigue are risks any time you add more decisions to your life, elastic habit decisions are smartly limited, intuitive, and easy to make. But be warned, if you go crazy and add six levels of success and five different habit options, you risk *both* choice paralysis and decision fatigue. There's a point of strongly diminishing (and then negative) returns when it comes to giving yourself options, so at least at first, stay at or below the recommendations in this book.

The Excitement of Variable Results

We've talked about the dangers and risks of choice, and learned how to limit them. But what about the upside of choice? Other than the obvious upside of being able to choose the option that works best for you each day, there's one other amazing benefit of a multi-level goal.

In casinos, the house always wins and you're guaranteed to lose money in the long term. So why would anyone be even remotely interested in that? How can people get addicted to gambling when it's basically just throwing money away?

If people can sit down at a slot machine, continue to push the spin button for hours, and lose money doing it, there must be something *powerful* driving their behavior. If I set up a booth that said, "Pay me 25 cents every time you push this button," I would get very little business, but this isn't too different from what a slot machine does. The key difference between them is variability.

Casinos utilize *variability of result* to keep people's interest. People gamble because when they put a dollar into the machine, it doesn't just spit out 92 cents every time. Instead, it uses a random number generator to create a wide variety of results, from a complete loss of that dollar to winning thousands of dollars and everything in between. Because players don't know what will happen on the *next spin*, they keep spinning, hoping for the big win. Variability keeps us interested and engaged, even in a surefire losing situation such as gambling.

Elastic habits introduce daily variability into habit building! If you're to pick something to get addicted to because of variable results, healthy habits are your best choice.

Chapter 8 Closing Thoughts

By carefully balancing stability and flexibility, we can maintain our sense of freedom while showing up consistently and generating powerful results. Increased stability reduces decision fatigue, while increased flexibility caters to our needs and keeps us engaged through the excitement of variability.

PART FIVE

Elastic Habits: Fully Applied

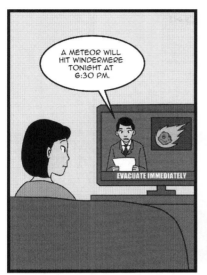
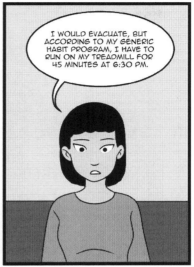
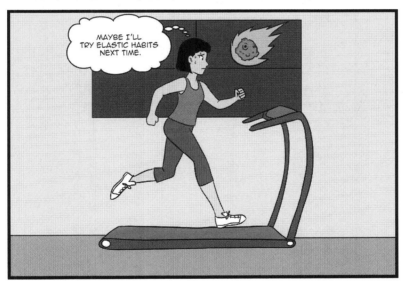

**Your elastic habits can adapt to your life
and (small) meteors.**

Chapter 9
Elastic Habits in Seven Easy Steps

"Winning is not a secret that belongs to a very few, winning is something that we can learn by studying ourselves, studying the environment and making ourselves ready for any challenge that is in front of us."

— Chess Grandmaster Garry Kasparov

Now you can apply all we've discussed, and create your own elastic habits! For this process, I recommend getting out a pen(cil) and paper to write everything down. The seven steps for shaping your behavior with elastic habits are as follows.

1. Choose (up to) three habits.
2. Choose (about) three lateral options per habit.
3. Choose (up to) three vertical targets for each lateral option.
4. Choose your cues and commit.
5. Display your habits.
6. Track your habits.
7. Score and evaluate your performance (optional).

Here's what one elastic habit might look like when it's finished.

Violin

Mini	Practice 1 minute	Study music 1 minute	Play 1 song
Plus	Practice 10 minutes	Study music 10 minutes	Play 3 songs
Elite	Practice 30 minutes	Study music 30 minutes	Play 6 songs

Violin is the elastic habit. Practicing, studying, and playing songs are the lateral options. Each of those lateral options has three intensities (Mini, Plus, Elite). Let's start with step one, choosing your habits.

1. Choose Three Habits

First, choose (up to) three general habits. You may choose fewer if desired. With any more than three habits, your energy and focus will be too diluted. And yes, you may be an exception, able to excel with six elastic habits, but if you have more than three elastic habits and struggle, it's because you have too many.

Goals such as *exercise* are generally too vague to be actionable. That's why people usually pick something specific such as push-ups, lifting weights, or running. But an elastic habit actually *needs to start out as general as possible*—specific actions are revealed as the habit stretches laterally (step two). An elastic habit's ability to represent multiple behaviors solves the awkward "Does editing count as writing?" type of questions that come from a specific goal such as "Write 1,000 words per day."

Because your elastic habits start broadly before narrowing to specific applications, you can see the bigger picture *and* its components. General habits represent the bigger picture goal we're trying to achieve.

- When people say they want to do 100 push-ups a day or run, they mean they want to get fitter, healthier, and stronger. *They generally want to exercise for its various benefits.*
- When people say they want to write every day, they also want to edit, brainstorm ideas, create outlines, and organize the structure of their books and articles. *They generally want to create and refine content.*
- When people say they want to meditate, they might also want to do yoga, use float tanks, or go on hikes in nature. *They generally want to practice calmness and mindfulness.*
- When people say they want to pull weeds, they might also want to plant, fertilize, and harvest their garden. *They generally want to garden.*

Use the broadest terms possible to cover multiple specific applications. Examples: garden, exercise, piano, woodworking (or even broader, crafting), creativity, cleaning, writing, relationships, mindfulness, healthy eating, reading, or any skill you want to build or area of focus (violin, juggling, soldering, engineering, home improvement, programming, public speaking, confidence, etc.), and so on.

Impactful and Values-Based Habits

I recommend choosing habits that can impact *multiple* areas of your life. Exercise is, in my opinion, the greatest habit because it improves your physical health, mental health, mood, energy level, perspective, and confidence. It even rivals prescription medication for fighting anxiety and depression.[1] The best habits have that sort of halo effect on your life. Another example: cleaning. When my home environment is clean, I get the side benefits of feeling calmer and being more productive.

Also try to choose a habit that connects with your values. If your habit is attached to something you care about, you'll want to do it. If you don't know what habits you want to choose right now or if you have so many options that it's hard to prioritize them, start with your values.

Write down your *current* top values. Life is full of different seasons, and what matters to you most right now might not always matter most to you. For that reason, be honest with yourself about what you really want and need in your life *right now* (instead of what you think you "should" value). My most important values right now are:

- Physical and mental health
- Honesty and integrity
- Creativity
- Freedom
- Learning
- Relationships

We want three habits maximum, so pick your top three values. Most likely, the values you think of first will be the right ones to focus on. But some of your values simply won't be as actionable as others. For example, honesty and integrity are extremely important to me, but they are already a part of who I am and are passively involved in the decisions I make; they aren't something I need to set aside time to "practice." So my top three *actionable* values are health, creativity, and freedom.

If you can't narrow down to three values, do this next step to help you see which behaviors are most attractive. From your values, identify general behaviors that would further your pursuit of them. Here are mine.

- Health: Exercise, meditate, eat healthy foods
- Creativity: Write, read books, experiment, brainstorm ideas
- Freedom: Earn money, manage money, invest in my career

Any behaviors derived from your values are prime candidates for your elastic habits. Looking at this list, you wouldn't be surprised to find that my elastic habits are exercise, reading, and writing. These three habits align with my values very well. Writing is particularly valuable because it connects with my values of both creativity and freedom (I can write any time and any place and writing earns me money).

Have you selected three general behaviors as your elastic habits? Great! It's time to stretch them laterally.

2. Choose (About) Three Lateral Options per Habit

In this step, you're going to think of the specific ways you want to pursue each habit that you chose in step one. There could be just one, or even dozens of ways to pursue something.

Before we get to specific examples, I want to mention that *time* is the universal lateral option. It works for almost any habit—spend X minutes doing a behavior. This can be especially useful for habits that involve too many activities to label (e.g., running a business or exercise). As you choose lateral options, consider if a "time spent" catch all is an option you'd like to have.

There are two downsides to using time spent as a primary measurement:

1. Time spent is not always the best measurement of progress. I've had one hour work sessions that were more productive than some eight hour work sessions.

2. Time may be too vague of a starting point. I know exactly what it means to run one mile, as it's a specific exercise with a clear stopping point. But "exercise for 20 minutes" is so open-ended that I have to convert it into a type of exercise before I begin. That extra step is enough of a hindrance to stop us sometimes. On the other hand, "read for 20 minutes" is just as straightforward as "read 10 pages."

Time is a universal measurement, and it can work well for many habits. But consider the downsides and how they might affect each habit. For writing, time is a poor metric compared to word count. But for reading, time works very well because pages/chapters of books vary wildly in size (and many kindle books have no page numbers). Thus, time is actually the most accurate measurement for reading progress (assuming you read for the entire duration).

Lateral option examples:

Drinking water (1 lateral option): If you want to develop the habit to drink more water, there's one behavior associated with that—drinking water. In this case, you probably won't have any lateral flexibility (but you'll still get vertical flexibility in the next step).

Reading books (1–3 lateral options): Reading is the obvious behavior here, but also consider researching and buying/borrowing books, as that's an important part of the reading process. Even so, my reading elastic habit has just the one option of reading. Just because there are multiple possible behaviors for a habit does not mean you need to utilize them all. Consider how each lateral option fits your goals and choose only the one(s) that work(s) best for you and the habit(s) you want to develop.

While reading is my only option, I give myself two ways to measure it—pages read and time spent reading. Sometimes, it's convenient to note the page you start and end at. Other times, there are no page numbers, and you can simply note the time you start reading. By having both as options, you eliminate possible sources of resistance ("This kindle book doesn't even have page numbers, but I can use time instead.")

Exercise (dozens of lateral options): There are practically infinite numbers of ways you can exercise. Dancing, sports, weightlifting, running, biking, hiking, pull-ups, walking, and yoga are all great ways to exercise.

You can write down everything that comes to mind. This is the one area where there's a lot more flexibility. You might have nine types of exercise that genuinely interest you. There's something called a habit pool that can work with large numbers of lateral options. But for most habits, and for the sake of keeping it simple, pick one to four options, with a general aim of three.

I've chosen exercise options that I enjoy and do most often. These don't necessarily exclude other exercise options; they just give me focal and reference points. The spirit of this system is flexibility, so even if Yoga isn't one of my "officially listed" options, I may choose to substitute it one day by comparing it to one of my official options. Or, of course, I can just set an "exercise X minutes" option for all of the unlisted ways I can exercise. Here are my current lateral exercise habit options:

- Gym (basketball or weights)
- Push-ups/pull-ups
- Laps around my neighborhood (walking or running)

Journaling (1–2 lateral options): Don't be quick to assume that there is only one lateral option for an elastic habit. In the case of journaling, you can review previous entries. If you're going to journal your thoughts about life, it makes sense to look back on what you've written in the past to learn from it and see how you've grown over time. Reviewing your journal entries can be an additional behavior that fits your journaling habit.

Writing (several lateral options): Besides writing content, you can create an outline or edit content. Editing itself has many different levels: developmental, substantive, copyediting, and proofreading. That is to say, the writing process involves a lot more than just writing, and only setting a word count doesn't take this into account. After you finish the first draft of a book, you don't need a word count goal, you need to edit! If you write for your career, you can add marketing as a part of your writing habit.

I recommend to aim for three lateral options per habit with a soft limit of four. More options are good to have, but only to a limit. At three, you'll have options, but it won't be too hard to decide between them. This is a balance of focus and flexibility. Fewer options increases focus and decreases flexibility. More options decreases focus and increases flexibility.

If some options are more "core" or important to the habit than others, that's okay. We can work with that in the next step.

At this point, you should have three general habits with one to four specific applications each. Next, we're going to add in the vertical flexibility that makes this strategy so much fun.

3. Set (Up to) Three Vertical Targets for Each Lateral Option

In this step, you're going to create one to three levels of success for each lateral application of each elastic habit.

Let's say you've chosen gardening as your habit. From that, you chose pulling weeds, watering plants, and general care (time-based) as your lateral options.

Since you're a gardening wizard, you know that your gardening needs may vary from day to day and week to week. There's composting, harvesting, weeding, planting seeds, transplanting, and more. This is where the flexibility of an elastic habit shines, because we can customize the habit for the specific reality of gardening. It's possible that, on some days, your garden won't need care. For this reason, we can make the Mini level a garden walkthrough. You can walk through your garden every day, and set Plus/Elite goals for days on which your garden needs care.

Gardening

Mini	Walkthrough		
Plus	Pull 5 Weeds	Water Plants	General Care (15 min)
Elite	General Care (30 min)		

Here's another example. To see the lateral options as discussed in step two, look across the top row. To see the vertical options of this step, look up and down each column.

- Elastic habit: Fitness
- Lateral options (four): sprinting, squats, timed exercise, gym
- Vertical options (always three): Mini, Plus, Elite

Fitness

Mini	1 sprint interval	10 bodyweight squats	Any exercise (1 min)	-
Plus	3 sprint intervals	40 bodyweight squats	Any exercise (10 min)	Show up at gym
Elite	6 sprint intervals	100 bodyweight squats	Any exercise (25 min)	Gym for 40+ minutes

You might be wondering where to set each target. What makes a behavior Mini, Plus, or Elite? Let's start with Elite.

How to Set Your Elite Targets

The Elite level gets its name from the fact that, if you did it every day, you would become elite in that area, or be well on your way to it.

I set this goal by asking myself, "What level of achievement would I be proud of the next day?" If you hit this level, you're going to feel really good about what you did. This is the size of many mainstream goals, but this time, it will feel infinitely better because you're doing it out of choice instead of an arbitrary commitment to a rigid goal. You're free to choose the easier Mini or Plus win conditions on any day, giving this more meaning when you do reach it.

Most of these are going to be sized at 30–60 minutes, though it depends on each person and habit.

If you want, you can make the Elite level seriously difficult. Since this is not something you have to do every day and it represents the highest level of achievement in this area, you can set the bar as high as you want.

If you set the Elite target extra high, then you're likely going to get more "Plus" and "Mini" wins as your bread and butter. Be careful, though, as it could be discouraging to set this target too far out of reach. I absolutely love seeing Elite wins on my tracker, and am encouraged as I get more of them.

Experimentation is encouraged!

How to Set Your Plus Targets

Plus is your mid-level target. The best way to think of this goal is something you'd deem "respectable." This is going to be 10–20-minute goal territory, where time is the best measure. My starting Plus goal for exercise was 25 push-ups or pull-ups (and has since increased to 35). I can actually complete those quickly, *but the amount of effort required is moderate*. Whether you measure by time or effort is up to you and can vary with each habit.

I set this goal by asking myself, "What level of action, if taken today, will make me think, 'That was good' tomorrow?"

You don't want this to be too small, or else it will swallow up your Mini goal. If your Plus goal is just a hair more difficult than your Mini, your Plus will essentially take over as your Mini, and then you'll basically just have two goal levels, one of them a larger-than-ideal minimum. You don't want this to be too large, either, because it will compete with your Elite goal and/or seem too difficult to complete often. The placement of your Plus goal is very important to maintain balance.

How to Set Your Mini Targets

Finally, you have the critical safety net, the Mini. Imagine this as scaling a mountain: you can try to climb to Plus and Elite levels near or at the top of the mountain, but if you ever fall for any reason, this net keeps you alive and lets you climb again tomorrow.

Make the Mini win condition *truly small*. One minute of activity is the recommended baseline for a mini habit. You have higher targets in Plus and Elite, so there is no reason to be ambitious here. A lot of people who read *Mini Habits* would talk to me or others about their mini habit of doing something for 10 minutes. That is about 10 times more difficult than a mini habit should be, and closer to Plus territory. Again, daily goals are personal to you and vary by habit, but 10 minutes is generally too high for a safety net for new habits.

Your Mini target needs to be something you can do *every single day without exception*. In other words, this net needs to be able to catch you every time, from any fall, from any height. This is absolutely crucial to your success with elastic habits. *You should be able to do this action on the worst day of your life.*

When your cat scratches your face in the middle of the night, your baby wakes you up at 4 AM, you're late to work (and your boss is a jerk), you find out your 12-year-old daughter got a tattoo last night, your energy is as low as your car's flat tire, and you have diarrhea ... on *that* day, you need to be able to meet the Mini level. *Easily.* Heck, days like that are why we *need* easy wins.

Some of my Mini options take less than 30 seconds. If I'm absolutely swamped, overwhelmed, depressed, and defeated one day, I can complete every habit's Mini level and be done for the day in less than five minutes. That's five minutes *total* for all three of my elastic habits, not each. Because I can win the day in under five minutes, I never lose.

While it's true that "mini" is relative to each person, anything over five minutes is outside of the expected range for something you can always do on your worst and/or busiest days. My editing Mini level is five minutes because I write for a living, so if you're already pretty invested and advanced in an area, a larger than usual Mini target might make sense.

I believe the real reason people have set too-high mini habits in the past was that they didn't want to have an embarrassingly small goal as their only option. I understand that, but now we have other options, so let's do away with the 10-minute "mini" goals and instead make them stress-free and small.

I tend to favor untimed actions for the Mini level because they're often easier and simpler, and don't require a timer. My Mini level of exercise started at three push-ups—I can do that in 10 seconds. Even if you do set a timer for an activity, you don't necessarily have to time it exactly. Just make sure you do it for at least the time you set.

If you want to use a timer for your habits and have smart home technology, it's very easy to say, for example, "Alexa [or other voice assistant], set a timer for one minute." And for a fun timer, you can do your habit for the duration of one song (songs average three to five minutes in length).

Proper Spacing Makes this System Hum
Once you've set your targets for each behavior, look at your spacing. Does each goal have its own space and appeal? If the Mini and Plus are too close, or the Plus and Elite are

too close, it will cancel out their unique benefits.

Clear separation helps us to mentally compartmentalize things. I lived in a one-bedroom apartment in Seattle that was 1,100 square feet—a good amount of space for one person—but it was just one giant room. All of the living areas blended together. This made it difficult for me to focus on work in my office because I was also in my bedroom and living room. When I moved to an apartment with separate rooms and doors (gosh, I love doors), it instantly improved my productivity and sleep.

If your Mini is one minute, your Plus should be something like 10 or 15 minutes. Plus goals should be somewhere around 3–20 times more difficult than a Mini goal. The Plus goal shouldn't intimidate you; it should range from easy-moderate to moderate. Elite goals are usually 2–4 times more difficult than the Plus goal. So if your Plus goal is 10 minutes, your Elite goal should be about 30 minutes.

How exactly you size each of your levels is, of course, completely up to you. Each person will respond uniquely to different targets, so experiment and learn what works best for you. This system has 15-day checkpoints, a good time to adjust your goals or keep them the same and try to do better in the next 15 days.

With color-coded tracking (we're in step 3, tracking is coming up in step 6), you'll see exactly how well or poorly you respond to your goals. My reading goal started out with almost exclusively Mini wins. That showed me that I needed to rebalance my targets. Once I rebalanced, I got more silvers (Plus) and even a couple of golds (Elite). This wasn't an arbitrary win that I got by reading the same amount as before and giving myself more credit for it. I actually read more pages and books because my revised goals were more enticing and reachable.

The Beauty of Self-Correcting Goals

This system is self-correcting. By analyzing your progress (or lack thereof), you can precisely tune your targets.

If you miss any days, it means your Mini goals are too big and too difficult. Make them smaller, a size you can't ever fail to do. This will solve your consistency problem and keep you going.

If you only get Mini wins, make your Plus goal smaller. The Plus goal is supposed to be "moderate," a fair distance from the Mini goal but still reachable. If you never reach the Plus level, it's a clear sign you should move it lower to make it more attainable and attractive.

If you get no Plus wins, but many Elite wins, it could mean that your Elite goal isn't hard enough and/or is too close to your Plus win condition. If your Plus and Elite win conditions are barely different, of course you'll go for the Elite win. That may not seem like a problem, but it is, because it basically eliminates your *crucial middle option.*

Let's use my lap walking/running option (part of my exercise elastic habit) as an example of balance.

- Mini: 1 lap (0.6 miles)
- Plus: 3 laps (1.8 miles)
- Elite: 6 laps (3.6 miles)

At these levels, the Mini option is a quick hit-and-run win that I can do in less than five minutes. If I want to reach Plus level, it's going to take me about 10–25 minutes to walk or run three laps. Then, if I want Elite, it's going to take at least double what I just did to earn Plus. It works well because there's enough space between them to make each option an enticing combination of effort and reward. I've found that, when I reach Plus, I go for the Elite win about 30–40% of the time. That's a sign of good balance, because it pushes me to greater wins, but also gives me satisfying middle-ground wins.

Can you guess the one issue in this example? The Mini is a little bit too close to the Plus. I rarely go for a Mini win here because: 1. my other Mini exercise options are faster and easier (10 push-ups, for example) and 2. if I take the time to go outside in running clothes, I'm almost always going to have the momentum and motivation to go at least three laps.

But even with this imperfect balance, this has been a valuable addition to my exercise elastic habit. If I went out there knowing I *had* to walk/run at least three laps, I probably wouldn't go as often. That's the power of freedom. Because I give myself the freedom to do only one lap, I show up and always do more. I don't think I've ever done only one lap to date, but the psychological freedom to stop there remains crucial to my success.

As you can see, even when your targets aren't perfectly balanced, your other lateral options will help to fill in those gaps. It's great to have multiple routes to each level of victory.

The Plus level is a good benchmark for properly balancing your targets. If you get, on average, a Plus win each day, your system is well balanced. You will have better days and worse days, but if that's the average day, you're good. A caveat to this, of course, is if you make your Elite goals so difficult that you're only getting Plus wins. That could lower your typical result and change the dynamic quite a bit.

- Mini goals should be extremely easy and laughable to miss.
- Plus goals should be a decent challenge, but nothing intimidating.
- Elite goals should be difficult, but also exciting when completed.

Ever since I started my own elastic habits, I've achieved more "Elite-sized" wins than at any time previously in my life. I get them regularly, because I have the potent combination of freedom and incentive. Many successful people and economies become so because they are incentivized and free to act.

We always have an incentive to improve our lives, but when it's packaged in a constricting and suffocating manner (as in every other strategy I've seen), we quit because our freedom is more important to us. Now you'll have more freedom than you've had in any goal or habit system you've tried before.

Elastic Habit Ideas and Examples

You can use these targets as guidelines for how to pick your targets and balance them. Don't pay too much attention to the specific numbers. I put thought into them, but these aren't customized to you. Pay more attention to how they're balanced and the strategic thinking behind their construction.

Fitness (Example 1)

Mini	1 sprint interval	10 bodyweight squats	-
Plus	3 sprint intervals	40 bodyweight squats	Show up at gym
Elite	6 sprint intervals	100 bodyweight squats	Gym for 40+ minutes

Fitness (Example 2)

Mini	Stretch 1 minute	5,000 steps	Dance for 1 song
Plus	Stretch 10 minutes	10,000 steps	Dance for 3 songs
Elite	Yoga for 30 minutes	15,000 steps	Dance for 6 songs

Fitness (Example 3)

Mini	20 jumping jacks	0.2 miles on treadmill	Go swimming
Plus	100 jumping jacks	1 mile on treadmill	Swim 10 laps
Elite	300 jumping jacks	2.5 miles on treadmill	Swim 24 laps

Healthy Eating

Mini	1 extra serving of fruit/vegetables	1 meal upgrade	-
Plus	2 extra servings of fruit/vegetables	2 meal upgrades	-
Elite	3 extra servings of fruit/vegetables	3 meal upgrades	Mega meal upgrade

A meal upgrade, which I introduced in *Mini Habits for*

Weight Loss, means making one small aspect of your meal healthier than usual. This means that, even if you're eating an unhealthy fast food meal, it's not the total loss you might think. You can choose to chew each bite 30 times, drink water instead of soda, drink a glass of water before eating, get a lettuce wrap instead of the bun, or swap your fries for a healthier side. To determine what counts as a healthy upgrade, use your past behavior as a marker. If you already always drink water, that's fantastic, but don't count it as an upgrade.

Example: Say that you're at a restaurant, and a burger, fries, and soda are what you'd typically get. You could do a lettuce wrap instead of the bun, coleslaw instead of fries, and water instead of soda. That's three meal upgrades for an Elite win, or do one or two of them for a Mini or Plus win, respectively. Alternatively, you could simply choose a healthier main dish (salad, salmon, etc.) to count it as a "mega" meal upgrade, an Elite win.

Drink Water		Read Books	
Mini	Drink 1 quart (32 oz.)	Mini	2 pages
Plus	Half gallon (64 oz.)	Plus	15 pages
Elite	Gallon (128 oz.)	Elite	40 pages

I recommend getting a half gallon or two-liter jug if you want to drink more water and track your intake. It's not unwieldy like a full gallon, but it still holds a lot of water and only needs one refill if you want to drink one gallon a day. If you do want to drink more water, just make sure it's spread out over the day and not all at once (water intoxication is dangerous).

As for reading, if you use an e-reader as I do, not all books have page numbers, making time a better aim in those cases. You could say either two pages or one minute of reading for the Mini level.

Gratitude

Mini	Write what you're thankful about for 1 minute	Reflect deeply on 1 grateful thought	Thank someone who isn't expecting it
Plus	Thankful writing 3 minutes	Reflect deeply on 3 grateful thoughts	Thank 2 people by person, phone, or email
Elite	Thankful writing 10 minutes	Reflect deeply on grateful thoughts for 15 minutes	Buy or make someone a thoughtful gift

This is a good example of how elastic habits can accommodate non-daily actions. If you went out of your way to thank someone every day, you might run out of new people to thank; it might feel forced if you thank the same people. That's why you have the option to reflect on or write grateful thoughts each day as your go-to action. But when you have an opportunity to thank someone meaningfully, you can give yourself appropriate credit for being grateful.

You can also highlight certain behaviors by making them the only option for a particular level. This is a very flexible system. Consider this gratitude alternative to the example above, and how it might change your behavior.

Gratitude (Alternative)

Mini	Reflect on your blessings (1 min)		
Plus	Write 300+ words of gratitude	Thank someone who isn't expecting it	-
Elite	Write 600+ words of gratitude	Buy or make someone a gift	-

Sometimes, it's better to have fewer options to narrow your focus and/or specialize in one area. You don't have to give each behavior full verticality. Just make sure that you have a viable daily option for each level. For example, buying or making a gift is a great Elite option here, but it isn't likely something you could do every day. But you could certainly write grateful thoughts each day.

Mindfulness

Mini	Meditate 1 minute	Yoga with focused breathing for 1 minute
Plus	Meditate 10 minutes	Yoga for 10 minutes
Elite	Meditate 30 minutes	Yoga for 30 minutes

Writing

Mini	Write 50 words	Edit 5 minutes
Plus	Write 500 words	Edit 30 minutes
Elite	Write 1500 words	Edit 2 hours

This is my writing elastic habit. It has worked very well. I don't always use a timer for editing. I often look at the clock when I start and don't always edit uninterrupted (distractions in the modern age are relentless). But I do get a good idea of which level I achieve. As for words written, my writing software, Scrivener, automatically tracks my daily word count.

Journal

Mini	Write 1 sentence	-
Plus	Write 1 paragraph	Write 1 sentence & review one week of entries
Elite	Write 1 page	Write 1 paragraph & review one month of entries

Woodworking

Mini	Spend 2 minutes on woodworking project	Write down 1 new woodworking project idea
Plus	Spend 20 minutes on woodworking project	Write down 5 new woodworking project ideas
Elite	Spend 1 hour on woodworking project	Design and plan a new project

Public Speaking

Mini	Diaphragm exercises 1 minute	Tongue twisters for 1 min. or 7 reps	Practice a speech 1 time
Plus	Diaphragm exercises 5 minutes	Tongue twisters for 5 min. or 25 reps	Practice a speech 3 times
Elite	Diaphragm exercises 10 minutes	Tongue twisters for 15 min. or 50 reps	Practice a speech 6 times

There are many, many more options for elastic habits, of course, but I hope these gave you some ideas.[2] On to step four!

4. Choose Your Cues and Commit

A traditionally formed habit has one cue to trigger the behavior; it's usually a time of day or following another action. I call these time-based and action-based cues.

Time-based cue: Do the behavior at a specific time. For example, brush your teeth at 8:45 AM.

Action-based cue: Do the behavior after a different action, usually an already established habit. For example, brush your teeth after you shower (I brush mine *in* the shower, which makes entering the shower my cue).

Traditional habit cues like these are fine to use. They work. If successful, you'll form a single-root habit that will eventually become semi-automatic. If you want to introduce something into your life that you don't have to think about much about and just do, this is a good choice.

The cue-behavior-reward loop explains how the habit process works in the brain, and it's where we get the idea for traditional solo cues. The cue creates the idea or craving to do the action, the action is done, and we experience some kind of reward from the action. The only problem is, *real life habits can have more than one cue.*

Using the Bad Habit Model ... for Good Habits?
Most bad habits have multiple cues. They're formed unintentionally and "in the wild"; they resemble an uncontrolled bamboo forest more than a contained houseplant. For example, you might smoke cigarettes socially, while eating, while drinking, while gambling, when stressed, when celebrating, and more. The wild, multi-cue bad habit stands in stark contrast to the way we are taught to form good habits.

Your brain's subconscious doesn't differentiate between bad and good habits—they're both processes that lead to a reward. Most people recommend a single cue to serve as the *only catalyst* for a good habit, but bad habits show us a new way, especially for personality types like mine.

My personality type is spontaneous and rebellious. The hyper-structured traditional habit doesn't merely disinterest me, it *repels me*. Some people like to have every day laid out in a schedule. I don't, and while I may be in the minority, I'm also not alone in that. I am not saying that anyone is right or wrong, as these *preferences* largely come down to personality type. And, to be clear, if you enjoy having things scheduled and want to form traditional single-cue habits, you will have *great* success with elastic habits (better than with any other habit formation strategy). I am, however, going to discuss their downsides and another option for people who want the benefits of daily habits without the monotony.

Rigid rules are great ... until they break. For all their benefits—being clear, simple, and streamlined—single specific cues can also feel restricting, robotic, and awkward (if you miss them). If you aim to meditate at 5:00 PM and you miss that cue for whatever reason, what happens next? You've missed your one and only cue. You've failed the mission. Do you just do it later? If so, why did you have such a specific cue in the first place? If you miss your "one shot," you might decide to just skip the activity altogether.

Bad habits are notoriously strong and difficult to get rid of because they have *multiple roots*. Someone who figures out how to stop smoking socially still does it when upset. Someone else figures out how to eat healthier lunches, but unhealthy night snacking remains a struggle. Can you imagine if you had a good habit with this sort of resilience?

It's not going to happen accidentally, and it won't happen with other strategies that don't acknowledge that we are capable of doing *good things* with more than one cue.

In some cases, for some people, and for some behaviors, it's ideal to have a single cue. Absolutely, this is true, but notice the exclusive nature of that language. There are *a lot* of cases, people, and behaviors that will work better *without a specific cue.* I introduced this idea in the original *Mini Habits* book with the "any time before bed" option. The "no cue" option turned out to be my and many others' favorite way to pursue habits, and it gets even better with the *Elastic Habits* strategy.

The Daily Cue (No Cue)
I use the daily cue for all of my elastic habits. With no specific cue, you dramatically increase flexibility. But, as we discussed in the last chapter, all flexibility with no stability creates a useless blob on the floor that can't move.

If you say, "I have to write 50+ words 30 times this month," you could meet your target 30 times *on the first day and be done for the month.* If you allowed that much flexibility, you'd undercut the daily stability that enables habit formation. That's why habit cue flexibility is always bound by the day at a minimum.

A cue can be almost anything—a thought, a smell, a sound, a person, another action, a feeling, a desire, a place, a time of day. Any and all of these cues can trigger the same behavior. The daily cue means that you're not choosing only one, but opening up to all possible cues.

If you choose the daily cue, you're aiming to complete your habit(s) any time before you go to sleep. This gives you the entire day to find a way to succeed, even if it's right before your head hits the pillow. It helps you plan out bigger wins, rest when you need to, and form habits with multiple cues.

While I resist the idea of being robotic and scheduled, I do love having daily habits as a flexible structure for my spontaneous life. I want to establish my identity as someone who writes, exercises, and reads books (my elastic habits). With a flexible daily cue, I do all three of these things every day, but in different ways, at different times, and in different quantities.

Daily cues are not as "automatic" and mindless as someone's morning shower habit, but they can be just as reliable, as I and thousands of others have proven with years of success using the original *Mini Habits*. What daily cues lack in routine, they make up for in improvisation, flexibility, and diverse roots.

A huge benefit of the daily cue is that it removes micromanagement. With specific, individual cues, you must assign one for every habit. But if you choose the daily option, you don't have to remember when and where you need to do which habit, you just need to do them at some point in your day.

Window Cues

Let's say you find the time-based cue too restrictive and the daily cue too unstructured. If you want the stability of a single cue with *some* flexibility (but not the full day), consider creating a window cue.

A daily cue is basically a 16-hour window of time every day (if you sleep eight hours a night) to get your habits done. A window cue is simply a narrower window of time to get one or more behaviors finished. It's usually an hour or two, such as after you get home from work until 8 PM. It's just like how the cable company says they'll be at your house some time between 9:00 and 11:00 AM (hopefully you'll be more reliable than they are).

Window cues could work very well for someone who tends to have the same "window" of free time each day (or on weekdays). If you know that your best opportunity to do your habits is always going to be after work and before another activity, consider making that your window for one or more of your elastic habits. You could even set up multiple windows, such as before and after work, but if you're at the point of managing multiple cue windows, you're probably better off just calling it a daily cue to include *all* of the various windows of free time in your day.

I like the daily cue because it automatically selects your window(s) of free time as the cue. When you come to a point of free time in your day, think about your habits. For changing lives and varying schedules, this can be a relief. But if you have a very predictable and consistent schedule, a window cue, time-based cue, or action-based cue might work best.

Flexibility Testing

More flexibility means more win conditions. That's why I recommend that people—unless they want or need to schedule their habits—begin with the daily cue. The daily cue fits the elastic habits system and ideology very well. But if that fails, try the window cue. If *that* fails, try a specific time or action cue.

The idea here is to give yourself as much flexibility as possible at first. Only reduce it if you find that you need more structure to get it done. This will come down to your particular lifestyle and how seriously you take your habits. If you take your habits seriously and commit to them, you will *rarely* forget to do them. I forgot to read *once* in my first three months with three elastic habits. That's one time out of 270 attempts.

If you do decide to go with a time- or action-based cue or the window cue, I recommend having a failsafe plan. If you miss your cue or window, get the Mini win so that you can fight another day.

You could develop the habit of marking and checking your tracker before bed to ensure you've completed each habit. In habit formation and in life, it's not about dominating every battle the same exact way each time; it's about always showing up and fighting the smartest fight in each situation.

The Morning Plan Cue

The idea behind elastic habits is to allow your daily goals to be adaptable to your life. Showing up in some way each day is everything when it comes to forming habits. Since life is crazy more often than not, there's no way to predict whether tomorrow will be like today, or that the situation two weeks from now will be the same as it was two weeks ago when we made our goals. Daily adaptability allows us to improvise to any and all internal and external conditions.

The daily cue, while it provides this benefit, isn't structured. This can be problematic for those who can't find a way to work their habits into their day. A good alternative between being completely flexible and completely structured is to create your plan each morning.

Morning is a great time to scope out your day and make plans for when and how you'll complete your elastic habits. You'll have a general idea of your other scheduled events and even an initial read on how you're feeling that day. This is far more information than most people are used to having when it comes to setting goals, as usually goals are predefined. Thus, the morning is a great opportunity to make an informed plan about how to attack the day.

You do *not* have to decide what level of habit you want to do today. But I would recommend deciding on which lateral option makes sense for you, and then doing however much of it you decide when the time comes. If you want, you can of course plan to do the Elite level of a particular habit, but I want to caution you to remain flexible if that doesn't happen for some reason.

The major pitfall of most goals is all-or-nothing thinking, where the person sees the big goal they originally planned isn't going to be met, and decides to do *nothing* instead. This system avoids that. While I encourage you to plan for and get those Elite wins, I also want you to be ready to get the emergency Mini win in case you don't get the big one.

Plans can change, even over a few hours. Be aware of that. With the morning cue, you'll make your plans in the beginning of the day, and, almost every time, I bet you'll succeed doing exactly what was planned. But never forget that you're unstoppable as long as you refuse the zero day. No detour should completely derail you.

Cue Recap

- **Daily (recommended):** Do the behavior some time before sleeping for the night. (Guitar any time before bed.)
- **Morning Plan Cue (recommended):** Every morning, set your elastic habit plans for the day. Choose a lateral option for each habit, and optionally choose what level of success to achieve. (I'm going to go to the gym at 7:30 AM before work, I'll do at least one mini upgrade at lunch, and I'll clean the kitchen tonight. That will satisfy all three of my elastic habits for the day.)

- **Window:** Do the behavior in a specific window of time. (Archery between 3:00 and 5:00 PM.)
- **Time-based:** Do the behavior at the same time every day. (Garden at 3:30 PM.)
- **Action-based:** Do the behavior immediately following another behavior. (Exercise after getting out of bed in the morning.)

Given the lateral elasticity of your habits (multiple behavior options to complete one habit), I recommend the daily cue, because the flexibility allows you to choose the cues *and* behaviors that make the most sense each day. Alternatively, you can pick a different cue for each lateral option as checkpoints throughout the day. For example:

Elastic Habit: Exercise
Lateral Options: Push-ups, Walking/running, Gym

- Wake up: Push-ups
- 12:30 PM: Walk
- After work: Gym

In this example, you have cues at multiple times in the day, and your goal is to complete one (or more) of them. Again, I believe this is best handled as a daily cue, because you can intuitively choose to do one or more of these when they are available. Micromanaging multiple cues isn't usually necessary, because the flow of your day, your energy level, and so on will make the right choice at the right time obvious to you. It's simply less complicated with daily cues.

The daily cue is the least structured, most flexible cue you can possibly have. That makes it like the human shoulder joint—flexible and powerful, but susceptible to problems if not properly cared for. To support the extreme flexibility of a daily cue, you need to rely on a very critical piece of structure. You need to commit.

Commit and You Will Succeed

Commitment is important in habit formation, regardless of how you choose to pursue it. If you don't commit to a behavior, you will stop doing it. I do my elastic habits every day because I'm committed to getting no zeros on any day. The only valid excuses I have to skip my habits are illness and vacation, two situations in which I don't require *anything* of myself. (I might still do them in those cases, but it's not required.)

Commitment is hard, I know, but this is different. It's *easy* to commit when you have complete flexibility in how and when and in what capacity you do your habit. The reason 30-day challenges are so prevalent and three-year challenges aren't is that *people can't bear to commit to follow them longer than 30 days.*

People often struggle with commitments because they're not sure they *want* to commit. Yet marrying someone is the biggest commitment a person can make, and people *celebrate it* as the best day of their lives. Commitment is joyous if you love what you're committing to, and you're going to *love* committing to elastic habits.

I had no problem committing to my elastic habits for life, because ...

1. They're fun: I can compete against myself. I can win in a variety of ways. I don't have to write the same monotonous checkmark or X every day, because every victory and reward is valuable, yet measured. I get a new score every 15 days. I can earn bonuses. Elastic habits are like a fun game that I can't lose (as long as I show up), and they benefit my life directly and significantly.

2. They're supportive: Your habits will shrink into

super-easy mode at any time, for any reason, and for any duration. I can decide to "take a whole month off" and just complete the Mini level of my three habits (less than five minutes a day). I won't get the same results or satisfaction as I do when I'm pushing myself more, but I will maintain everything about this system that makes it powerful—showing up every day. I can push myself on my terms now, based on the changing situations and circumstances of my unique life.

3. They're exciting: You know the part in *King Kong* where he beats his chest? I hesitate to put this on public record, but I've literally done that multiple times because of this strategy. I feel like that on many days. I know exactly what that gold Elite sticker represents, and it's *thrilling* every time I earn it. In the past, I would feel good about big wins, but not *this* good. I would feel encouraged, but not *this* encouraged. That little gold sticker is proof that I crushed it today, and I can look back on it any time if I forget how far I've come. Unlike other habit formation strategies, elastic habits tell a story about your journey to greatness; it's easy to document, quantify, and review your wins and progress.

If you choose the daily cue, commit to it. Every day. Take it seriously. Never forget your easy safety net (the Mini level) if you can't do a habit earlier in the day. Do that, and you'll go far.

5. Display Your Habits

I highly, highly recommend that you display your habits in your home. You can go ahead and burn your habit journal now, because this isn't something to be hidden in secret. Decisions like these can be the difference between failure, success, and extraordinary success.

If you want to do this the right way, you'll need to display *two* things.

1. Your elastic habits
2. Your habit tracker

Regardless of how you *track* your daily habits (the next step), I recommend writing down your elastic habits separately to put next to your tracker. Why? A typical elastic habit has *nine* win conditions, meaning it isn't going to fit into a small space.

Instead of "Run one mile every day," you have nine options of different fitness activities and intensities to choose from. This elasticity needs to be large, appealing, and easy to see and process.

I created specialized products to make this system work seamlessly, but they aren't necessary for success—you can do this using materials at home. You can simply type and print your habits on regular paper, or write them on (colored) notecards and place them in a grid. Then, when you want to change them, you can edit your document, print out a new sheet, or write on a new notecard. Let's talk about tracking.

6. Track Your Habits

Most habit-tracking systems require an X or a checkmark, because there is only one level of success. We have three levels of success, meaning we need three different kinds of notation. We don't want just any notation, because there's an important psychological principle at play—prioritize consistency and reward all levels of success *as successful*.

In order to prioritize consistency and reward all levels of success, I recommend using only subtle differences in notation as you increase your level of success. Don't use a real diamond to mark an Elite win and pin a dead fly to your wall to mark a Mini win. They are both solid, valuable wins! I'll use the official elastic habit tracker as an example of how to approach this.

Color Coding and Marking

Some people use color-coded stickers for different habits. For example, blue stickers for drinking more water and orange stickers for cleaning. This is an insult to the purpose of color coding! Your habits already have their own row and name to identify them! They don't need their own color, too. We can use color to differentiate our levels of success.

The official *Elastic Habit Tracker* is designed for 3/8" colored round stickers (both are sold at minihabits.com). After you complete a habit, *use the colored sticker that corresponds to the level you did* (green for Mini, silver for Plus, and gold for Elite). The stickers are the same size and shape, suggesting they are equal "wins" in many ways.

Note: If you are color blind, you may be able to differentiate shades of differently colored stickers. If that is too challenging or if you don't want to use stickers, you can also use symbols to represent the different levels.

If you use symbols, I suggest one of the following progressions. Why? Because a key benefit of using stickers is iterative success and these symbol progressions allow for that. At any point, you can upgrade from Mini to Plus, Mini to Elite, or Plus to Elite.

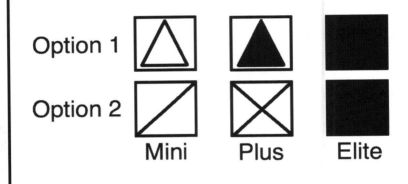

Iterative Success

If you use a marker and mark your box green for Mini, but later in the day you unexpectedly get Elite, well, your box is already green with no easy way to change it (while wet-erase markers work on the official tracker, I don't recommend erasing one color to write in another).

Using stickers, you can simply put the gold sticker *over* the green one to replace it. Similarly, the triangles and squares are iterative sequences that allow you to add to your current win if desired. Start with a triangle for Mini, color it in for Plus, and then color in a square (or circle) over the triangle for Elite. It's important to allow for iterative upgrades in your notation because it leaves you with the opportunity to get surprise upgrade wins, which I can assure you are inspiring and delightful occurrences.

If you want to use a standard calendar, you can use stickers or symbols on the sides, top, or bottom of each day's box to correspond to your elastic habits. For example, make fitness the top left, reading the middle left, and voice training the bottom left. It's not as clean as the official tracker and lacks the scoring component (covered in the products chapter), but it has the advantage of integrating into your current calendar.

It takes about 20 seconds to fill in your three habit boxes with a sticker or symbol each day. That's the only "daily maintenance" this system requires!

What about Mobile Apps?

Depending on time, money, and demand, it's possible I'll create a mobile app for tracking elastic habits in the future (no guarantees). But this is a good time to mention that physical habit tracking is almost always superior to virtual tracking.

Apps are much like thoughts, in that they can get lost in the competition with thousands of other apps on your device. While most people carry a phone with them at all times, their convenience is offset by the fact that they are distraction hubs. I've never had lasting success with mobile habit tracking apps, but I have had remarkable success with real-life calendar tracking because it's never forgotten or lost in my digital world. I've had more success than I've ever had before using the elastic habit tracker I've created—I don't miss days and I regularly get Elite-level wins.

I understand that we live in modern, tech-heavy societies.

But that's a good reason to put your habits into the physical world where they can stand apart. There's something about tactile interaction and tangibility that makes paper habit tracking more satisfying and "real." Seeing your progress on paper also makes it feel more official. (College diplomas aren't digital for good reason!)

All that being said, the other reason I've never had success with apps is that they're not designed for smart and strategic habit strategies, just basic ones. As of this writing, there isn't an app out there that can support the lateral and vertical flexibility of an elastic habit. To try to track an elastic habit in a standard habit tracking app would be a royal mess, but you're welcome to try.

If you have requests or suggestions, send me an email at stephen@minihabits.com.

7. Score and Evaluate Your Performance (optional)

Elastic habits have three levels of success. This opens up a whole new level of tracking. In most systems, people just check yes/no for doing their habits; now you can quantify your performance for each habit and each day. You're still going for 100% daily victory as with any other strategy, but you can also keep an eye on how often you rise above and beyond the minimum.

Tracking your elastic habits with the official tools takes no more time or effort than tracking a standard habit. The scoring component of *Elastic Habits* is optional, however, so if you want, you can simply track your success and not use scoring.

This Is Easy

This system might seem complicated as you read through this, but that's only because I'm explaining the strategy behind it, which is advanced. If I explain the inner workings of a computer, and why it's put together in a certain way, it will sound complicated, but the end product is intuitive, easy to use, and powerful. Case in point, for all of these options we've discussed, it takes only 20 seconds a day to maintain this system! This is how easy the system is in practice.

1. You can pursue three habits at a time.
2. Each habit is flexible, with multiple options at multiple intensities to fit your day.
3. You just need to complete your habits at some point before you go to sleep for the night. (Otherwise, you can define cues for each behavior or some behaviors.)
4. Display and track your habits each day. I've created tools to make this as easy as possible: A Habit Poster clearly displays your habit with all of its win conditions. The Tracking Calendar makes tracking your success enjoyable.

Once you've chosen your habits, defined their lateral and vertical flexibility, and set up your habit tracker, this is the easiest and most rewarding system ever. You will look at your habit poster, decide what to do at what intensity, and mark what level you reach on your tracker. I'll mark a habit right after I complete it, before I go to bed, or the next morning.

All you have to do to maintain this system is mark three boxes each day. And in return, it gives you a stable yet flexible structure to maximize your days and make progress at a pace YOU customize. I'm not going to tell you when to get an Elite win—you are going to decide that for yourself. I'm not going to tell you when to slow down and take a break with some easy Mini wins—you are going to decide that for yourself. Every person is different, and this system effortlessly accommodates the unique flow of any and every life.

To put it succinctly, an elastic habit is just like a normal habit, except that you have *several* ways to win (each with their own advantages) instead of one. More win conditions means more wins. Different possibilities each day means less boredom with the process (a common habit killer). Next, we're going to discuss advanced tactics, and how to succeed every day.

Chapter 9 Closing Thoughts

While countless hours of thought, experimentation, and research went into the design of this strategy, the end result is a simple, low-maintenance, and streamlined way to build habits and achieve short-term results. While this system takes only seconds per day to maintain, it gives you powerful incentives and great satisfaction for daily successes of all sizes.

Chapter 10
Advanced Strategies and Tactics

"Recognizing the need is the primary condition for design."

— Charles Eames

The following strategies are optional and more advanced than the core *Elastic Habits* system that we just covered. They offer a plethora of customization options for those who desire it.

Modular Habits

We can do some fun things with the verticality of elastic habits. The default, assumed way to measure vertical success is with iterative reps of any behavior.

Iterative Reps Examples:

- Writing: 50 words, 500 words, 1,500 words
- Exercise: 5 push-ups, 30 push-ups, 100 push-ups

By default, the next level of success is gained by doing more of the same behavior, while different behaviors are used as lateral options. But with a modular habit, additional behaviors become the *vertical component*. Let's use cleaning as an example. People use their kitchens every day to prepare food. You could use this modular habit for cleaning the kitchen. To get an Elite win in a modular habit, you must do *all three* behaviors (or just do one for the Mini).

Kitchen Cleaning (Mod)

Mini	Dishes and Sink
Plus	Counters Wiped and Cleared
Elite	Floor Swept and Mopped

The sink and dishes are the heart of the kitchen. If those are in disarray, the kitchen is borderline unusable. Therefore, doing the dishes and cleaning the sink could be your first (Mini level) option for kitchen cleaning. The Plus level is organizing the counters and wiping them. And finally, the Elite level is cleaning the floor.

Here's a modular habit example for fitness (again, this is just one of your three lateral options for fitness):

- Mini: 2-minute stretch routine
- Plus: 10-minute calisthenics video
- Elite: 10-minute "Ab-wrecker 3000" video

The routine flows together, but if you stop at any point, you still benefit from it. At the Mini level, you get a nice stretch. At the Plus level, you get a stretch and a small workout. At the Elite level, you've completed a full 20+ minute workout.

For modular habits, make the Elite level easier to do. Unlike a standard elastic habit, the Elite level of a modular habit includes *all three actions,* and therefore the higher-level actions shouldn't be as difficult as usual.

Musical instrument:

- Mini: Practice chords 1 minute
- Plus: Practice a song 15 minutes
- Elite: Study music theory 15 minutes

If you complete the Elite level, it's 31 minutes total since it includes every action in the column.

Saving money:

- Mini: Make coffee at home
- Plus: Bring lunch to work
- Elite: Make dinner at home

Public speaking:

- Mini: Diaphragm exercises for 3 minutes
- Plus: Tongue twister reps for 5 minutes or 20 reps
- Elite: Practice a (2-minute) speech 5 times

Modular habits are great for multi-skill practices such as public speaking. You can work on your vocal power with the diaphragm exercises, enunciation with the tongue twisters, and poise with speech practice.

Interchangeable Habits

Modular habits are done in order. Interchangeable habits are done in *any* order. To give you an idea of what this might look like in practice, here's an example of a full cleaning elastic habit. It includes a modular habit, an interchangeable habit, and two others.

Cleaning

	Kitchen (Modular)	Quick Clean Up	Misc Cleaning	Deep Cleaning (Modular, Interchangeable)
Mini	Dishes and Sink	1 Room	1 Minute	Vacuum
Plus	Counters Wiped and Cleared	2 Rooms	10 Minutes	Dust
Elite	Floor Swept and Mopped	3 Rooms	30 Minutes	Scrub Bathroom

While it looks like a lot of options, choosing each day is simple. Simply start with the type of cleaning you want or need to do (the top row in grey), and then look at that column's options.

The first column, kitchen cleaning, is modular, meaning it must be done in that order for each successive level. The deep cleaning behaviors in the final column are modular *and* interchangeable, meaning you can start with any of the behaviors, such as dusting, for a Mini win.

As you can see, by making some elastic habits modular and interchangeable, you can accommodate *almost any desired combination of behaviors*. Your cleaning habit can encompass multiple types and levels of cleaning to fit the diversity of ways you clean your home.

Adding modular capability to the core elastic habits concept brings an explosion of creative potential to designing your habits. You don't even need to limit your modular options to three.

Habit Pools
Since the vertical component of a modular or interchangeable habit is a matter of picking one behavior at a time from a pool of options, you can consider having up to about six modular options in your pool (before it gets too cumbersome). Each completed behavior in the pool

represents a level up.

For all interchangeable habits, it's important to try to make them about the same difficulty. And for reference, you should size them at roughly Plus level or slightly smaller. Since these are all worth one level up, you don't want to make them too big or too small.

Exercise pool example: 15 pull-ups, 20 push-ups, 30 jumping jacks, 30 bodyweight squats, one mile run/walk/jog, 10 minutes of stretching

Do any one for Mini, any two for Plus, any three for Elite!

Elastic Routines

An elastic routine is a string of behaviors done in succession. These are different from typical routines because you can choose the *intensity* of the routine (Mini, Plus, Elite) each day based on your available time, motivation, and energy. They are vertically flexible, but not laterally, because the behaviors are predetermined.

I recommend a maximum of five behaviors for your routine. Here's an example of a four-behavior morning routine. Morning routines are the most likely choice, but you can also create bedtime routines or midday routines.

Morning Routine (Complete Any Row)

	Step 1	Step 2	Step 3	Step 4
Mini	1 Push-up	5 Bodyweight squats	1 Yoga pose	Brush teeth
Plus	10 Push-ups	25 Bodyweight squats	3 Yoga poses	Brush and floss
Elite	30 Push-ups	50 Bodyweight squats	5 Yoga poses	Brush and floss

You can see each routine by looking left to right, going across the row. The mini routine is one push-up, five bodyweight squats, one yoga pose, and brushing your teeth. Consider these other ideas for your morning routine: any daily grooming or hygiene activities, writing, reading, preparing breakfast, planning your day, meditating, exercise, meal prepping, email replying, "phone fasting" or not using your phone until a certain time, getting up by a certain time.

The difference between an elastic routine and a modular habit is that a routine must be done in its entirety at a chosen intensity, while a modular habit can be partially completed. A routine is more difficult than a single elastic habit or modular habit because it requires multiple behaviors, but it's a great value for the effort because the actions are streamlined together. These are superior to standard routines because you can vary your intensity by the day. For example, if you don't have much time in the morning, you can quickly do the Mini routine.

I recommend that you count one elastic routine as *two* elastic habits because it contains multiple behaviors. Thus, my recommendation of three habits maximum would allow for one routine (worth two) and one habit. But it also depends on your goals and how difficult you make the routine. Since these behaviors are done in succession, you won't have very much friction *between* the behaviors, making a routine of three to five behaviors only marginally more difficult than a single habit. Starting is the hardest part, but once you're moving through the routine, momentum will help you finish it.

I recommend giving your elastic routine a specific cue (not the flexible daily cue). Since an elastic routine of three to five behaviors is relatively large, even at its smallest level, it needs more structure than a regular elastic habit does. A regular elastic habit works so well because it allows you to plan for big wins on some days and fit in smaller wins on other days. But bigger, more elaborate habits and routines require more planning to succeed consistently, even at the Mini level, so pick a time or action to trigger the first behavior of your routine.

The morning routine cue is easy and automatic—waking up is the cue for action. You get a structured cue without even having to think about it! That's why the morning is the perfect time for routines; if you start with a set of assertive self-care actions, you'll notice a big difference in your day. Elastic routines give you an answer for rushed days, relaxed days, stressful days, and everything else!

Just remember, you must complete ALL of the Mini, Plus, or Elite actions to earn that level. If you prefer, you can use a modular habit for a morning routine, which would take away the requirement to do every single behavior.

Changing Targets

All of the most successful companies in the world use data to improve their processes, services, and products. You can now do the same with your habits! If you make a change, you'll be able to quantify exactly how it affects your performance. Changing your targets should only be done for two reasons:

1. The number is way off what it needs to be.
2. The end of a 15-day period or month has arrived.

The reason you want to wait until the end of the period, if possible, is to standardize your results. If you start out with one set of targets and change it halfway through the period, then your results will be harder to interpret. If you keep your targets the same, you can see how you performed *with that particular set of goals* that period or that month.

If you want to use the first 15 days as a test period, you can adjust your targets frequently as you learn what works for you. If you want to change targets but are still curious to evaluate your current set of goals, wait until the end of the 15-day period to change.

Sprints

In *Elastic Habits*, there exists a magical idea called a sprint. We know what "sprint" means in running, swimming, and even in goals, so why is this different?

The most common goal-based "sprint" people do is a 30-day challenge. They try to drastically change their behavior for 30 days. It's not bad as an experiment, but it's also not great as a personal transformation tool. Thirty days is arbitrary and has no scientific merit. It's better than nothing, but it's not as good as it can be.

The major problem with goal sprints is that they *end*. Once a goal sprint ends, what do you do? Not much! That's when you gradually or swiftly go back to who you were beforehand. There's almost never an *after* plan, and that reminds me of a wise saying that goes, "failing to plan is planning to fail."

The *Elastic Habits* framework is unique in that it can stretch in *any way*. It can accommodate "sprint challenges" very easily within its natural framework, without interrupting your overall habit-forming trajectory. Importantly, you already have a plan in place for *after* your sprint (your normal elastic habits), and you even have a plan in case your sprint goes poorly and you need to quit for whatever reason. You always have the safety net of "I'll just do the Mini today." No matter what, you will make progress every day.

You can take on challenges at any time in your journey if you want to spice it up. I recommend you keep them to 15 days or less, especially because you get to score yourself after 15 days. That's one more great benefit of doing sprint challenges in this system—you already have a scoring framework in place to document and reward your sprint. Here are a few sprint ideas ...

- Elite sprint: See if you can go three days in a row with Elite wins in *all* of your habits.
- Perfect week: See if you can get seven Elite wins in a row for one of your habits.
- Power play: Try to get Plus or higher in all of your habits for an entire 15-day period.

If you decide to pursue a challenge, never forget that it's within the framework of the *Elastic Habits* system. And that framework says that you need to at least get the Mini win or higher every day. Do NOT let an Elite miss become a complete miss, because then you're at risk of losing momentum and falling into the same all-or-nothing pattern that kills most habits and goals. Grab the Mini win and try again tomorrow, or regroup and retry the sprint challenge at a later time.

As for why these challenges are any different or better than other challenges, it's because you get to push yourself in a *completely safe environment.* If you fail one or more days of your challenge, you can still pick up the Mini win later in the day to avoid the dreaded (and costly) no-show. These challenges are different because you aren't going all-or-nothing; you're going for a big accomplishment with an even bigger safety net to catch you if you miss.

Snowboard Lessons: Safety First for Maximum Progress

I went snowboarding for the first time in my 30s, and my hips are tighter than Warren Buffet's breakfast budget. That combination doesn't exactly translate into a successful outing, or at least it didn't for me. I struggled mightily and switched to skiing, which they said was easier. Well, shucks, I was terrible at that, too.

I was in a group of about 10 people. We were all doing our own thing and occasionally going down the slope together. But I had a huge problem as a beginner—I couldn't slow down. It seemed that, no matter what I did, I blasted down the hill at full speed. Somehow, I would go *faster trying to brake* than people who *weren't trying to brake*. It seemed like a prank, as if someone had glued powerful magnets at the tip of my skis that were attracted to a supermagnet at the bottom of the hill.

Since my hips rotate about as well as the one bad wheel on a shopping cart, my early braking attempts ended up bringing my skis closer together without digging into the snow enough. If you watch the pros at the winter Olympics, they bring their skis together when they want to go *faster*, and I think I was accidentally doing that. *Sigh.*

With poor steering and max speed, I was basically a human snowbullet. I would frequently fall down on purpose ... to save lives. I even feared for the forest. I could have easily killed a tree (I know).

My friend, who had been snowboarding a couple dozen times before, went down the slopes with me one time and saw how defeated I was (in every way). We reached the bottom of the slope, which required skiers to slow down and bank to the right into the lift to go back up the mountain. If you kept going straight, there was a long gravel area to unceremoniously "slow you down," which somehow seemed worse than going down the entire mountain.

My friend told me to waddle back out and ski on the gentle slope coming in to the lift. He looked at my technique, trying to figure out my braking problem. He told me to squeeze my thighs together and put my skis in a position that looked like this V flipped upside down or a pizza, but I had limited success.

The following story is 100% true, down to the timing. After going 0 to 60 mph instantly a few more times on the gentler slope, and seeing small children casually carve snow with ease, I said in frustration, "Ugh! Why am I the only person here who can't slow down?" I pointed at the very next guy coming down the hill. "Here, this guy," I said, "watch how effortless this is for him." We both watched this man come in fast, not slow down even a little bit, and go head over skis when his first ski hit the dreaded gravel area. It looked like a cartoon. "Okay, bad example," I said as we laughed.

Thankfully, the man was okay, but it was one of the funniest things I've ever seen, especially because I randomly decided to use him as an example of how easy braking was for everyone else. I could have actually taught that guy some stuff, like how to fall gracefully in the snow before reaching the gravel.

The Breakthrough

My friend was a hero to me that day, because he stayed with me in the boring lift area for about 45 minutes helping me out. And I finally had a breakthrough! I figured out how to dig my inner ski edge into the snow, and I *actually slowed down*. I still wasn't perfect but I made some progress, which made the rest of my trip significantly less life-threatening and a lot more fun.

Lesson: You can make great(er) improvements when you have a safe environment in which to experiment and learn. I made very little progress starting out at the top of the mountain. I would get to an unsafe speed (for my skill level) too quickly and have to bail out, leaving me less time to learn.

The encouragement from my friend and the gentle slope made me feel safe, which allowed me to focus on skiing instead of surviving, and ultimately resulted in my breakthrough. In the same way, elastic habits are nonjudgmental, accepting of all progress, beginner-friendly, and a fantastic springboard from which to launch yourself to greater heights. It's not because they push you until you front-flip into the gravel; it's because they are safe, and supportive of your every imperfect attempt.

Safe, Supportive Systems (SSS)

Safe and supportive systems are rare. Typically, you're asked to push yourself to your limits, all the time, every day, no excuses. This is fine in theory but problematic when, you know, you're an imperfect human being on one or more of those days.

People don't become great through sheer brute force; they become great through *training*. It's the *only* way. Here's the nuance: A select few are able to use brute force to train themselves, but most of us are some combination of uninterested and unable to do that to ourselves (going back to the freedom thing). Thus, alternative ways to train are warranted.

In a safe, supportive system (SSS), you can train on your own terms, never giving up your autonomy or freedom. Think about what the mountain did to me at first. It said, *you're going to learn going 300 mph or you're not going to learn at all.* That's why I kept falling and wanted to quit. I wasn't able to learn what I needed to learn in those conditions.

But the slope near the lift *was so mild that my friend had to push me to get started as if I were a child on a swing.* Did I really just put that information in my book? My editor, Carolyn, will remove it. [ed. note: Surprise!] While being pushed on the baby slope was embarrassing at first, it allowed me to focus on my technique and experiment without fearing for the children around me (superior little skiers, they were) or going into the mysterious and snowy forest.[1]

Chapter 10 Closing Thoughts

The Elastic Habits framework affords a number of creative possibilities. The strategies in this chapter are optional.

Chapter 11
How to Succeed Every Day with Elastic Habits

"The people heard it, and approved the doctrine, and immediately practiced the contrary."

"Well done is better than well said."

— Benjamin Franklin

My exercise elastic habit has four lateral options: push- or pull-ups, going to the gym, timed exercise (anything), or laps around a nearby lake. On the lake path, I can walk, run, jog, or interval train. Any speed is fine, as I count laps for success. It's 0.6 miles per lap, and my elastic habit levels are one lap for Mini, three laps for Plus, and six laps for Elite.

The Power of Showing Up: The Rain Run

One day, I didn't feel like doing much, but I figured I could run three laps to get a Plus win. Respectable. The previous time I went, I did interval training. This time, I decided to try running all three laps (1.8 miles). I was successful, but I live in Florida and it was over 90 degrees. So I decided to take a cool-down lap, walking slowly along the path with my water bottle. After that lap (#4), I liked the peaceful scenery and felt good about turning a lazy day into a good run. At that point, I realized I could leverage my momentum and get a *huge* win on an otherwise down day, so I decided to walk two more victory laps to bring me to six laps total (Elite win).

Note: If you complete an elastic habit at the Mini or Plus level and mark your win on your tracker, that doesn't have to be the end of it. You have until you go to sleep to upgrade any of your wins. I will often plan on reaching a certain level for each habit each day, but sometimes I'll change my mind and say, "You know what? I can do better than that, and I will."

Right after I finished my fifth lap, it started raining. Hard. Others on the path scattered home, but I stayed, because I needed to complete one more lap. While taking that final lap and getting soaked, I smiled. I felt like the storm represented all of the adversity in my life, and I kept moving forward despite it. I felt like a champion in that moment, knowing that I had earned a truly Elite win.

Before having elastic habits, I would have been upset at this storm. I would have thought, "Great, the one time I decide to run, it rains me out," before going home. But since I needed one more lap to achieve my ultimate victory, the rain didn't feel like a nuisance or sign of bad luck; it felt like a pitiful obstacle trying (and failing) to get in my way. I *laughed out loud* and raised my arms in the air like a runner who crosses the finish line in first place. (Don't worry, nobody saw this crazy fool in the rain because they were all indoors.)

Hard rainfall is epic in itself, but I felt like I was the protagonist in a movie. I think I know why. In all stories, protagonists always meet with an antagonist whom they must overcome, but never without reason. Protagonists always want something specific (a safe world, survival, career success, a love interest), and antagonists stand in their way.

Having specific objectives positions you as a protagonist (because protagonists always have objectives), so any obstacle that arises intuitively appears as an antagonist that you must defeat. When I eclipsed five laps, that sixth lap was the ticket to my Elite win. That's what I wanted. This is opposed to the much worse perspective *"I'm trying to get in shape and, wow, just when I finally got motivated to run, it starts raining."* See the difference? Specific objectives, especially when tiered, are powerful perspective changers.

Because of how my elastic habit framed my actions, the rain actually *enhanced* my experience and made me *more proud* about my accomplishment. This is the sort of magical moment that can happen when you have specific, tiered, elastic daily goals. In my experience, it happens a lot. You know you'll get at least the Mini(mum) win every day, but you don't always know how or when you'll do much more than you expected. Those surprises are as much fun today as when I first started.

I thought the *Mini Habits* strategy was as much fun as it could get, but this strategy is easily three times more fun. *Easily.* Instead of generic "bonus reps," you can quantify and celebrate specific levels of overachievement. And you can fine-tune your targets to encourage specific outcomes. It feels amazing, even in the rain.

My rain run was only made possible by my dedication to do

some form of exercise every day and fill that box in my habit tracker. It's not a difficult or heroic requirement, as I can complete it with three push-ups in under 10 seconds. It is, however, a smart and savvy strategy that puts me in a winning position every single day. It's exactly what every coach attempts to do—put the team in a position to win. More often than not, a team that has every opportunity to win through preparation and strategy will win. The same applies to us.

Elastic habits will put you in the most advantageous position you've ever been in. You'll feel completely free with lateral and vertical flexibility, you'll have tempting upside wins, and you'll have the silver bullet of consistency (the Mini win) to keep you in the game no matter what. As long as you continue to show up and at least meet the Mini requirement, you literally can't lose, but you can definitely win and win big.

The Mini Day

There is a great danger in underestimating or undervaluing the humble Mini win. I've written three books largely based on the impact of this small daily victory, but it remains the humblest in appearance of the elastic habit options. It's never going to grab your attention and desire as its larger counterparts can.

Make no mistake, the Mini level of elastic habits is the low-key linchpin of the entire system. Your ability to snag Elite win after Elite win is supported by your ability to actively "rest" on any previous or subsequent day with an easy Mini victory. The moment you devalue the Mini victory because you deem it inadequate is the day the whole thing falls apart.

I know the perfectionists out there will want to get that A+ every time. And to that, I have a very important distinction. The A+ in this system is not Elite. Elite is a sub-ranking. The first grade you get is either an A+ or an F, and it's determined by whether you show up (A+) or don't (F).

I recommend that, at least one or two times, you meet only the Mini requirement for all of your habits. That's three green stickers on your tracker. If you really want to do more, go ahead, but at some point, there will be a day in which it makes sense for you to quickly get the Mini wins and call it good. Once you do this, and see that you can get a fully winning day with such little effort, it will open your eyes to the full power of *Elastic Habits*.

I can't possibly overstate this, because all of the people who fail with this system will be those who discount the importance of the Mini level and choose to leave their tracker blank instead. That blank will lead to more blanks until they fall off completely.

The power of *Elastic Habits* is in the name—it's the total range of wins you can obtain without breaking your intention to act in these areas. Remember, elastic means *resilient*, especially while being stretched. If you ignore the Mini level, your habit will *shatter* when you need that smaller win to keep going. Allow your habit to flex in all directions, and it will be resilient to life's hardest punches.

Most of us are already familiar with ambitious goals and know their merits. Doing an "all Mini" day will help you understand that it's okay to have slower, less productive days sometimes in the scope of your long-term plans.

You might feel pressure to get at least one Plus or higher or even an Elite every day. Don't. Be *fully* flexible. Allow your habit to stretch in all directions and you will thrive at a level you never have before. Trust me, by accepting the "all Mini" day and letting it be enough, you will virtually guarantee your ability to stay on track for *life*. Unlike 30-day plans that literally tell you the day (#31) when they fizzle out and you gladly regain your freedom, you can practice this system successfully for *decades*. It will bend and flex and expand to your every need, to your every motivational burst, and it will grow with you!

How to Handle Vacations

It's my opinion that habits can be optional on vacation. The purpose of vacation is to experience something outside of your daily life. That said, I will sometimes modify my habits to be vacation-friendly.

There's no wrong decision here, but it's important to make a decision. For me, if any part of my day is a vacation day, I can take that day off. This includes the day I leave and the day I return.

Vacations options (from most strict to least strict):

- Require the same habits on vacation as at home.
- Modify your elastic habits to be simpler and easy to do on the road (perhaps a standard mini habit would work best here).
- Require elastic habits if you're home for *any* part of the day, but not if you're away.
- Give yourself a number of vacation days off per year from your habitual requirements and use them how you please (similar to how companies give vacation time).
- Exempt any vacation or travel day from elastic habits (even if you're home for part of the day). I mark these days with black stickers.

I've also created travel tracking cards, sized as regular business cards but designed for tracking your habits on the go (see them at minihabits.com).

It's absolutely possible (and not a bad idea) to continue your elastic habits while on vacation. It depends on your goals, lifestyle, and chosen habits. Whatever you decide, just make sure that you do decide, because if vacation comes and you have no process in place to deal with that, it could derail you. As Scar says in *The Lion King*, be prepared.

Pre-Pay Habits before Vacation

If you know you're going on a trip, you can make a deal with yourself to do extra on the day(s) leading up to the trip to count for the days you'll be gone.

You can't clean your home while on vacation, but you can clean a bit extra before you leave. Achieve the level you want for today, and then achieve an extra level to sub in for a day or days that you're gone. You could even do a marathon cleaning session to count for a full week or two of vacation (since a clean house is the goal, and you won't be messing it up on vacation, that works well).

If it's something like reading or writing, you can certainly do more of that ahead of a trip also. Most of the time, habits are seen as something to be done daily so that the neurological pattern sticks. But, thanks to their ease and flexibility, elastic habits are reliably done even before neurological assistance, so you don't necessarily need to worry about continuing the behavior while on vacation. You can simply resume when you return home.

But the other factor here is the scoring system. I took a four-day trip toward the end of the month, and I didn't want to get a zero score for those days, even though I'm allowed. So on the days preceding the trip, I did extra Mini-level accomplishments to count for those vacation days. That way, I got the satisfaction of maintaining a decent score for the 15-day period and month, and yet, I didn't have to worry about doing anything on vacation.

Intraday Perspectives and Strategy

If you choose the daily cue for your elastic habits, here are a few approaches you can take for getting your habits done. Most likely, you'll use a combination of these (as I do), but it helps to have some ideas.

Surprise attack: Quickly complete the Mini level of all your elastic habits. This takes away the worry or pressure. Then, consider taking any or all of them to the next level at some point during the day. The danger here is complacency, as you might be tempted to "get it done" and move on. I find it's better to consider each habit individually, but you might prefer this way. The times I do this are usually when I know I have a super-busy day ahead of me and can't think of a good time window to do my elastic habits. This way, I can knock them out early and worry about doing more later if I have the time and energy.

Context-driven: Look for opportunities to work your habits into your day. You can read on your phone just about anywhere. You can do push-ups just about anywhere. You can meditate anywhere, too. Some habits can only be done at home with special equipment, but many others can travel! It's good to know which habits can be done anywhere and which need a certain context.

One at a time: Some people like to do things in sequence. I'm one of them. I like to focus on one habit until I've done what I want with it. With this perspective, you can complete one elastic habit to any level, and then focus on the next one. I tend to prioritize writing and exercise first, and then read at night.

Plan it out: Even if you choose the daily flexible cue, you can still pick a specific time to do your habit(s) on any given day.

Combination: In practice, I use a combination of these strategies to complete my elastic habits each day, and you likely will, too.

How to Choose Intensity

You can do whatever intensity you want for any habit on any day. That said, it may be helpful to use something like this to keep your expectations realistic. If you don't know what intensity to choose, use the following guideline:

First, rate yourself in these three areas.

- Energy 1–10
- Free time 1–10
- Desire/Motivation to do the habit 1–10

Once you have a rating for all three, add up the numbers. If you get a score of 20+, go for Elite. If you get a score of 14+, go for Plus. Anything less, go for Mini.

Random Chance Decision with Dice

It can be fun sometimes to let the dice decide your fate. You only need to roll one. Before you roll it, be clear about which of your habits the roll applies to. Or if you desire, you can roll it three times and then "allocate" the three results to each habit.

1 or 2: Mini level
3 or 4: Plus level
5 or 6: Elite level

Promise that you'll do at least what you roll. You can also create fun variations, such as the one below giving you a bonus reward for rolling one or six.

1: Mini + Reward (food, movie, night out, etc.)
2: Mini
3: Plus
4: Plus
5: Elite
6: Elite + Reward (food, movie, night out, etc.)

If you're going to incorporate random chance outcomes into your daily habits, it's a good idea to add in random rewards. As stated previously, variability of result is known to hook us on not-so-healthy things like gambling, and here we can use it for our benefit.

Generally speaking, good habits are hard work to sustain at first, which is why perception is so important. When I play basketball for more than two hours, my body works as hard as it ever does. But I look forward to playing because I perceive it as an entertaining game instead of an arduous task. Elastic habits make habit pursuit fun from the start, and, by adding in something like this, we can improve upon that even further.

Exceptions into Rules: Using Reverse Exceptions

I heard a story of a man who was offered dessert on a dark

and stormy night. He looked outside and said, "Tonight seems mysterious and special, so I'll get the peanut butter cheesecake." Does this story shock you? Or does it sound like default human behavior to always find a reason for cheesecake?

We make exceptions all of the time. The problem is, the exceptions we make are often against our ideals.

- I'll gamble just one more $100 bill.
- It's the 8th of February, so I'll eat ice cream instead of fruit.
  - (Sub exception) That was delicious. Why not have just one more scoop? Just this once?
- I'll skip my workout tonight and get back on track tomorrow.
- Since I'm with friends, I'll have another drink.
- Eating doughnuts for breakfast every morning could be detrimental to my health, but doing it just this once isn't a big deal.

Exceptions are rarely harmful if they are truly exceptions—I'm not trying to shame you for eating a doughnut. But since exceptions bypass our defenses easily, they are likely to be repeated whenever our subconscious wants something. This combination can create issues.

The problem occurs when exceptions repeat so often that they become rules. If you find a reason to eat dessert after dinner more than half of the time, it's no longer an exception; it's a disguised *rule* that you will eat dessert.

I don't know of any smokers who decided they would be long-term smokers the first time they tried a cigarette. *I'll smoke a cigarette since I've never had one before* is the first exception that evolves into an addictive rule.

Reverse Exceptions

We've all experienced the power of exceptions in our lives, often to negative effect, but the reverse exception technique is a wonderful tool to help us make positive choices! It's called that because it's the reverse of how we typically use exceptions.

Here are some examples of how you might use reverse exceptions.

- I'm tired and wouldn't usually do anything active right now, but just this once, why not do a few bodyweight squats? Done. Now, I'll just run in place for 30 seconds. Easy!
- That cake looks good, but I'll just eat some delicious fruit this time instead. I can always have cake later.
- The TV is right there and I want to relax, but I'll just do the dishes quickly first. It'll only take a minute.
- I feel like ripping his head off right now, but just this once I'll spare his life and take a few deep breaths instead.

"Just"

You'll notice the heavy usage of the word "just" in the above examples, and that's no coincidence. Words carry powerfully influential connotations, and "just" has a very casual and nonthreatening vibe to it. That's why salespeople use it so often—for today only, it's just $999.99!

"Hmm, that's *just* $1,000? Maybe it's not overpriced."

Use self-talk like "just this once" when you're making reverse exceptions. It's counterintuitive to claim that it's good to only do a healthy thing "this one time," but we've all seen exceptions turn into rules over and over again, and it's no different with healthy behaviors. Make as many beneficial exceptions as you can, and you might see those exceptions turn into life-changing rules.

Exceptions are so vital to life because we're always making them. We're frequently torn between different options, and exceptions are often the tipping point. If you can get into a habit of making healthy exceptions, you'll be surprised at the positive impact it has on your life. Exceptions are known for prolonging bad habits, but they can help you lean toward better behaviors, too.

Overcome Resistance at Any Time

If you ever resist taking action, go through this quick process. It will work *every time*.

1. Confirm the ONE activity you want to do.

Many times, we face resistance to action because we haven't narrowed our focus to an actionable level. We know we can't do multiple things at the same time, so even if we have one thing we think we should do, as long as the other options are in mind and under consideration, we won't do it.

In order to take action, you must first terminate deliberation. When we make decisions, first we deliberate (weigh our options), and then we implement (act). But before implementation is possible, *we have to stop weighing our options.*

Ask yourself, "Am I still deliberating between options, or have I chosen one?" Until you can answer this question firmly with *one* action you'd like to take, you won't be in a position to succeed. If an action will benefit you, do it. Trying to do the perfect action in the perfect way at the perfect time is the enemy of action, and action is the foundation of progress and success.

2. Shrink your chosen activity until it's a simple mechanical action.

Forward motion is always the right answer, and the easiest way to move forward is to focus on the mechanics, not the concept. Let's say that walking is the action you've chosen, but you feel resistance. Resistance in this case comes from the baggage your mind attaches to the entire process of taking a walk. You might feel like you need to walk a certain amount to make it worthwhile, or you might feel strength-sapping shame from not walking enough in the past. Or maybe you're just tired.

Whatever the specific source of resistance is—there can be many—the solution is to shrink the behavior. This shifts your focus from the heavier concepts of the action to the simple mechanics of doing it. In order to walk, you place your left foot in front of your right foot, and then your right in front of your left. It's such an irritating and condescending sentence to read, I know, but that's why it's so important. It's a *joke* to think about the mechanics of something we've done our whole lives because it's beyond easy to do. When we feel resistance, "beyond easy" is the way forward.

The human mind is extraordinarily powerful, and resistance to action is one instance in which that backfires. We can (over)analyze everything, trip up on our own psychology, and forget the simplicity of walking, or writing our thoughts down, or making a call, or vacuuming, or lifting weights. When it's not a problem of overthinking, it's a problem of preexisting habits coaxing us to stay the same. The solution: If you're losing the mental battle, stop fighting and simplify. Focus on the mechanics, because they always work.

3. Once you've begun the behavior, the game changes.

Starting is the hardest part. Once you've started, you gain access to a whole new bag of tricks. You can set mini goals. You can challenge yourself. You can bargain (if I do this much work, I can play this much later). All of the motivational tricks and tools people try to use before action are *much* more effective *while in action*. Why?

Being in action is proof that you've terminated the deliberation phase. Even if it's a small step, your likelihood of doing more surges once you begin. I've found myself watching TV shows, commercials, and YouTube videos that I actively disliked just because *I felt I should finish them.* We've all probably finished watching movies we don't enjoy. In fact, I've only ever walked out of one movie theater (*Indiana Jones and the Kingdom of the Crystal Skull*).

As ridiculous as it sounds to continue doing something you dislike, it makes sense, because continuing your current behavior is almost always the path of least resistance. This same concept helps us do beneficial things that we resist doing. Pick one action, identify the simple mechanics of moving forward with it, and you'll be moving in a new direction *with momentum.*

Overcoming Resistance Recap

1. Resistance to action is first an issue of *clarity*: Have you chosen one objective you want to pursue right now?
2. Then it becomes an issue of *complexity*: Have you simplified the action to a mechanical starting point that is both clearly defined and easy to do?
3. Finally, it's a matter of *continuing*: When you take the first step, you're in motion. Once in motion, you

will find your efforts more successful than they were before motion. You can repeat these steps as necessary if you get stuck. The more you practice it, the better you'll get at it.

The Key to Commitment

It's one thing to commit. It's another to deliver on that commitment. About half of people who commit their lives to one another in marriage get divorced. Given the importance and weight of *that* commitment and its poor success rate, it's no wonder goal commitment has an even worse track record.

Have you ever had a package delivered late, even though the carrier or sender promised it would be on time? That shows us that commitment isn't the finish line; it's the starting line. When someone makes you a promise, your first reaction is not, "Oh good, it's done." Rather, you will instinctively evaluate that person's (or company's) trustworthiness. Trust is the foundation of commitment.

Self-Trust

How can you trust yourself if you've failed at reaching your goals for many years? Think about what it would take for you to regain trust in *someone else* who had lost yours. To regain trust in anyone, including yourself, you need *real evidence of change.*

Once trust is damaged, it requires success to overcome it. One success isn't enough, of course, as you need to repeat the pattern many times to overwrite the failure(s) in your memory. Successful repetition builds self-trust and new habits.

Here's where it gets tricky. You need self-trust to sustain a commitment, but real self-trust can only be earned by fulfilling commitments, creating a closed loop. This is why mini-sized actions remain the ideal base of a behavior change strategy. They're easy commitments to fulfill, helping you build self-trust and keeping you from losing it.

Trust is lost by breaking a commitment; it is gained by meeting a commitment. This is the case regardless of the size of the commitment. The greatest amplifier of trust is how consistently you fulfill commitments, not how big they are.

This is nothing new; it's ancient wisdom. The first part of Luke 16:10 says, "He who is faithful in a very little thing is faithful also in much."

Commitments are always a risk/reward proposition. If you fail, you lose self-trust (risk). If you succeed, you gain self-trust (reward). But it's not a 1:1 comparison, because one broken commitment damages trust far more than one success rebuilds it. This is easily seen in relationships, where even one single betrayal can ruin a relationship founded upon decades of loyalty. This naturally points us to small, easy commitments as the better option if given a choice, and indeed, this is the line of thinking from which *Mini Habits* was born. But *Mini Habits* was a little bit too conservative, for one reason.

The problem isn't that we commit to larger goals. It's that we're forced to maintain the same commitment when circumstances change. Larger commitments do give us a stronger sense of accomplishment, fulfillment, and self-trust when completed. Therefore, it's actually smart to accept a large commitment when you know you can and will complete it.

You may or may not be a world beater on your first day

with elastic habits, but you will certainly improve your self-trust every single day. Your winning streak will include a variety of wins, from Mini to Elite. Peppering in those larger-commitment wins will accelerate your sense of self-trust.

The brilliance of this system is that you don't ever commit to a particular level of achievement, but you will still feel you did (and gain self-trust as if you did) when you accomplish it. You're only committing to doing *something each day.* You'll make intraday commitments based on the texture of your day, which are fresher and easier to fulfill than stale commitments you made months ago.

Three Phases of Elastic Habits

There are three general phases in *Elastic Habits*. Don't take these timeframes as law, because timing will vary from person to person. If a strategy recommends that you do something for X days, that generally means it's too boring or too difficult to do for longer, or maybe not rewarding enough for you to say, "I could do this every day for a long time." Elastic habits can last you a lifetime because they are fun, exciting, and rewarding.

I'm telling you these three phases so that you'll have them in the back of your mind. You might realize one day that you've moved on to a more advanced phase of habit pursuit and greatness. This is what a healthy progression with elastic habits should look like.

Phase 1: Building a Foundation (Months 1 and 2)

Your first objective for forming any habit is consistency. You need to show up in some capacity every day. The Mini level practically guarantees your ability to do so, while the Plus and Elite level give you a fun and concrete short-term upside.

I've found the upside of the larger goals critical to help me stay engaged and interested, because, while small goals are excellent for maintaining consistency, they aren't very exciting. Unlike my experience with mini habits alone, I've remained excited about elastic habits *months into my journey*. That's what variety and stretch goals can do.

When you first begin, you will likely get a variety of different results, ranging from Mini to Elite. The exact number of each is not as important as proving that you can show up every day. First, go for consistency. Don't tweak your behaviors unless necessary. Don't be anxious to scale everything up. Once you've proven that you can show up, you can begin looking at performance in phase 2.

Phase 2: Stability and Refinement (Months 2– 6)

As you move into the second phase of building elastic habits, you'll begin to notice patterns about your behavior. You might notice that Sundays are worse than Tuesdays for your habits. You might notice that you go on short bursts of inspired Elite wins followed by Mini wins. You might notice one habit is much weaker or stronger than your others.

About two months in, you'll have proven that you can show up every day. You'll have gained enhanced stability, since your neural pathways will have changed in some way and you'll have built a good foundation of self-trust. At this point, you can look to make more strategic changes to your targets as you see fit. Tweak your strategy to suit your lifestyle or to encourage specific behaviors.

In this phase, with the refinements you've made, you'll stop worrying about showing up every day, and gain confidence that you'll not only show up, but do well when you do. Don't put a time limit on reaching this level; just be thankful when you get here, because it's even more fun!

Phase 3: Mastery (Months 6–12 and beyond)

If you make it six months to a year with great consistency in a behavior, you'll reach the *inflection point* of mastery. You won't have mastery yet, but you'll have reached the stairs leading directly to it. Here, you can, if desired or necessary, begin to shift your goals to a new aim of *mastering one or more of your elastic habits*. This will likely entail creating more challenging Mini, Plus, and Elite goals or trying to get more consistent Elite-level wins with your current objectives.

This is the phase many people try starting at, and that rarely works out well. Don't rush to get here. It will be obvious when you arrive.

If you reach this phase, you should be getting Elite level wins with regularity (about 50–75% of the time, depending on the nature of the habit). Now you can narrow your focus, get stricter with your requirements (reduce lateral options if you want to specialize), and push yourself a bit more. But there are a few caveats to this.

As you approach mastery, be careful with your Mini-level goal. As your safety net, this level needs to stay *very easy for you*. If you feel like you've begun to master a behavior, you might be tempted to increase your Mini requirement. That would be a mistake, because the Mini requirement is not meant to push you, even in advanced stages. That's what the Elite level is for, and to a lesser degree, Plus.

Say your Mini level starts at reading two pages in a book

per day. After a few months, if you find yourself reading two books a week from an average pace of 60 pages read per day, you're clearly crushing it. You might increase your Mini requirement to five pages in that case, but don't make it 30 pages. That's asking for trouble when something unexpected happens and you end up with a zero for the day. The Mini is a safety net and a spark. Don't make it a challenge.

As I've increased my fitness toward mastery levels, getting consistent big wins, I have increased my Mini requirement. All the way back in 2013, I started with a mini habit of one push-up per day, and I probably would have failed if it had been two. When I started my exercise elastic habit, I made the Mini level three push-ups or pull-ups. As of writing, it currently stands at 10 push-ups or pull-ups for Mini, which has been no problem for me to meet, even on tough days.

This is the only reason to ever increase your Mini requirement: Push-ups and pull-ups have become so easy for me that doing 10 today feels like doing one did in 2013. If I miss even one day because this number is 10 instead of three or one, I will decrease my Mini target. **Only increase you Mini level as your baseline proficiency increases, not to push yourself.**

Reactivity and Proactivity with Elastic Habits

Some might look at this system or my pathetic snow-skiing story and say, "This just encourages weakness. If you always adjust your goals to circumstances in your life, you'll never become great. You must push through obstacles to win." This perspective, however, misses the whole point of elastic habits. I know where this thought comes from.

Reactivity is responding to stimuli in your environment. If you're reactive, it's assumed that you will be passive *until* something gives you a reason to act in response to it.

Proactivity means you *cause* things to happen with no external input necessary. It means that *you're the stimulus* in your environment.

It's evident that proactivity is generally superior to reactivity because it lets us control the direction of our lives. But there are times for each. There's nothing wrong with being reactive to your circumstances and environment. In fact, if a car is about to crash into you, you need to *react appropriately* to save your life. Reactivity only becomes a problem when it is the primary driving force in your life.

Most goals do not allow for *any* reactivity. They simplistically look at the positives of proactivity and take a firm "proactive behavior only" stance. They suggest that you ignore any and all circumstances. This is admirable in one way, but profoundly stupid in another. Consider the car example in the previous paragraph—*it's extremely useful to be able to react.* Another great example is in sports—great players are known to proactively exert their will on the court or field, *but they also react precisely to game events.*

To maximize your potential each day, you need to be both reactive and proactive. The *Elastic Habits* system gives you the perfect way to utilize both of these concepts. Your habits flex up and down and sideways, meaning you can maneuver through life's challenges *and* be proactive about doing your best in every situation. This system doesn't hold anyone back from being their best—it simply supports us better than other systems do, helping us be our best and never punishing us when our best is below an arbitrary threshold. Having support isn't weak; it's the real prerequisite to greatness. Look at anyone who has done something great or received a prestigious award—they almost invariably talk about the support they've had which enabled their success.

The Nature of Elastic Habits

The *Elastic Habits* strategy is founded upon flexibility. And while I've shared the framework and modifications you can make to it, that doesn't mean you can't innovate upon it further. Maybe you'll come up with a better way to handle vacations. Maybe you'll figure out a brilliant reminder system.

As vast as the possibilities are, you can see that the nature and purpose of this system is to prevent failure. When I say failure, I don't mean having an off day or even missing a day. We have ways to remedy those! When I say failure, I mean long-term failure, where you give up on your goals and habits for a sustained period of time. That's what keeps people stuck where they are.

Those who are able to move forward every day, whether it's crawling a few inches or leaping to new levels, are the ones who change their lives. This system will empower you to be that person.

Chapter 11 Closing Thoughts

When the right perspective meets the right strategy, great things happen. This chapter focused on the right way to think about and approach your elastic habits.

Chapter 12
Conclusion

"Notice that the stiffest tree is most easily cracked, while the bamboo or willow survives by bending with the wind."

— Bruce Lee

To start the book, I laid the groundwork for habits that seamlessly morph themselves to fit your life. We've just covered the specifics of how to make that happen. Now, let's recap everything from a bird's eye view.

Ultimate strength and success are made possible by empowerment through freedom and flexibility. Too often, we rely upon self-slavery to rigid, pre-set standards that can't fit our dynamic lives. This creates significant frustration, tension, and procrastination. Eventually we quit in order to regain our freedom. By giving ourselves more freedom and flexibility to attack each day in the right way, we can build a very powerful and stable base for any behavior.

By limiting our flexibility to three habits with three applications each and three vertical levels of success, we mitigate issues like decision fatigue and choice paralysis. At the same time, we give ourselves the freedom to be the commander of each day, rather than following strict orders from a person or program that can't see the battlefield of our lives. With a plethora of weapons to choose from and nine times more win conditions than before, we're going to win a lot more often, because we finally have the tools to succeed in *any* life situation.

Varied options and multiple win conditions will keep us interested in the short and long term. Every day is a new opportunity to set a new personal best, or to take an active rest day if wanted or needed. You will never be punished for getting a Mini win, only rewarded for your consistency. You also have the option for greater rewards and satisfaction in Plus and Elite wins.

As we make progress over time, we can adjust our targets. Depending on your specific goals, you can maintain your sense of progression and challenge yourself with small, incremental increases each 15-day period, or you can try to master your current level before increasing your targets, or something in between. It's up to you!

The most important thing you need to do is track your daily completion of each habit and decide on a way to mark the level you achieved. I recommend color coded stickers, as the official tracker is designed to use. Or you can use a symbol progression method to allow for upgrades (in case you mark a Mini win in the morning and achieve Plus later in the day). I caution against something like "1, 2, and 3," because it gives the Mini level an inferior appearance. When a Mini win is the only win you can or are willing to achieve on a given day, it's the *biggest possible* win. Thus, it's not a good idea to imply that it's inferior, since it's actually the best sometimes. Each level has a place in your habit journey and life. Use them all and you will learn to love and appreciate them all!

Scoring is a fun (but optional) addition to the official habit tracker. It allows you to see exactly how well you did for each habit, each 15-day period, and each month. You can compare your scores to see if you're progressing, maintaining, or losing ground. Mini, Plus, and Elite wins are worth 1, 2, and 3 points, respectively. While I cautioned against using "1, 2, and 3" for tracking, it's okay to use use these values for scoring because it's done for analysis after the period is completed. There are also various bonuses to reward you for consistency, big winning streaks, and the number of Elite wins you get per habit or per period.

By putting all of these features into a low-maintenance system, you can win consistently on multiple levels, and you'll be able to do it for a long time.

Questions and Answers

Q: How do I pick the *right* behavior today if I have several lateral options?

The unique makeup of each day will often guide you to the best choice. But you can also set one or two preferred options for each elastic habit. Try to list them roughly in order of preference on your habit poster (or wherever you write them).

My preferred exercise options are weightlifting or basketball at the gym. I'll do walking/running/push-ups/pull-ups on rest days or especially busy days. Weightlifting and basketball align best with my fitness goals. The others are less aligned with my fitness goals, so I use them as second-tier options.

I've had plenty of stretches where I mostly do second-tier options. For example, I've had issues with "jumper's knee" from playing basketball, which makes jumping painful, but I can still walk or even run. Other times, my shoulder gives me trouble, making heavy weight training difficult, so I'll do push-ups or pull-ups as lighter conditioning work. And let's not forget the flexibility of elastic habits—I don't have to go to the gym even when I'm perfectly healthy and rested. It's *because* of that freedom that I so often choose to go.

You might be worried about not doing enough because you have the freedom to take the easy win. But you'll find that by tracking your behavior, you'll be more honest with yourself about when you're slacking. In any other system, slacking would bring on shame, but in this one, you can self-correct without all of the unnecessary baggage.

It will take some time to adjust to this. Many of us are used to being coerced—by ourselves, our goals, or others—to do things that don't match our situation. Even when we're capable of performing at a certain level, it can drain us to feel forced into it. Taking action from a place of freedom and personal power is a wholly different experience. You might have an unimpressive start or unimpressive streaks because you're so used to relying on outside pressure. But as you learn how to leverage your freedom, your power will emerge and your ceiling will rise higher and higher.

The greatest thing about this approach is absolute sustainability. If you're 100% free, there's no risk of ever having to quit. We quit things to regain freedom from their grip on our lives. This is why you can do good things if coerced to do them, but *great* things through personal freedom and empowerment.

Q: What if I miss a day?

Even as the creator and biggest fan of this system, I forgot to read one night. As I said in *Mini Habits*, missing one day is no problem, but two days in a row is a serious concern.

There's a study that shows one missed day has no negative impact on habit formation. But do not miss two days in a row if you can help it, as that sets a new trend in the wrong direction. I try not to miss even one habit on any day, because the momentum from winning every day is really powerful and worth fighting for.

If you miss a habit on any day, it's possible you just forgot, but it's also a red flag that something might be wrong. The first thing to look at is your Mini goal. Is it small enough? Ask yourself why you didn't do the Mini to get the win. If it's something like the Mini goal being too large, shrink it down to a level you can't possibly fail to do. If it's simple forgetfulness (like my case with reading), just make up for it and "patch it" and continue your journey ahead.

If you use the scoring card attached to the Official Elastic Habits Tracker, there's something I call a "patch" that can cover up a missed habit; that's what I used when I forgot to read, and, just like that, it was like I never missed a day. It's important to have a psychological recovery tool for honest mistakes like this. Nobody will be perfect. This system lets us make progress despite mistakes. If you patch a day, you won't have to look at the blank spot and feel bad about it. (The patch is further explained in the Elastic Habit Products section at the back of the book.)

Q: Why can't I have eight elastic habits?

Elastic habits stretch out laterally and vertically to give you freedom and power in areas that matter to you. They're not a way to do 8,000 things at once. In the next section, I will tell you an alternative elastic system for pursuing several behaviors at once in case you're interested. It isn't for building habits, but it is a fun way to pursue more behaviors.

If you really want to form habits, choose no more than three. That's still three times more than the one-at-a-time requirement for most other habit strategies. And, in my experience, you can make major progress in all three areas at once. Transforming three areas of your life is more than enough to improve it dramatically!

Q: When should I mark my tracker?

There are four times to mark your habits complete:

1. Right after completion
2. When you've completed all of them (and can mark them all at once)
3. Just before going to bed
4. When you get up the next morning

I usually mark one or two of my habits as done throughout the day, and check them all before I go to sleep. Ideally, we would never wait until the next morning to mark our habits complete for the previous day, but I've done it many times and it works fine. My poster is right outside my bedroom door and I can do it on my way to the kitchen.

There is only one instance in which I ever mark a behavior *before* it is done. If I am headed to bed and am going to read before I fall asleep, I will sometimes put a Mini (green) sticker in the slot. If I end up reading more than the Mini level and getting to Plus, I can upgrade it in the morning. But generally speaking, never mark a behavior before it's done unless you're going to do it immediately after marking it.

Look at your elastic habits every morning when you wake up. You don't have to decide everything in the morning, but you should have a rough idea of what behaviors you're going to choose today and, optionally, what level you want to reach for each one. If you do that every morning, you can also check to make sure that you've marked all of the habits you did the previous day.

Alternate Strategy: Elastic Actions

If you have a lot of behaviors you want to pursue and don't necessarily care about forming ironclad habits in any of them, there's another option for you.

Elastic Actions

Elastic actions are just like elastic habits in their setup—they have lateral and vertical flexibility. The difference is in commitment and habit formation. Elastic habits require daily commitment to form habits and solidify a behavior's role in your life. But elastic actions don't require you to do them at all. You can do them whenever and to whatever extent you want on any day. You can skip any actions or even full days.

The upside to the elastic actions plan is absolute freedom and a greater selection of actions to choose from. The downside is that you miss out on habit formation (which is a big deal!). Not all behaviors, however, are suited for habit formation. For example, you might not want to or need to tend to your garden every day.

The purpose of elastic actions is to raise your awareness about behaviors of interest and to reward you for doing them. You can still use the scoring system in the elastic habits tracker, which gives you an incentive to do more behaviors to a higher level more often. See if you can beat your high score!

If you really want to pursue six behaviors right now and can't narrow them down to three as suggested for elastic habits, try starting out with an elastic actions strategy. The official elastic habits tracker has room for six options. You'll see which behaviors stand out as ones you'd most like to build into your everyday life, and then you can switch to elastic habits with your favorite three.

The Fourth Month Epiphany

After multiple revisions of the habit posters and habit tracker, I had finally gotten it right. I had deliberately slumped at the beginning of the year to test this idea that I had been writing about since the year before. But when I realized the profound effect that little nuances in the tracker had on my motivation and performance, I knew I needed to refine it. May 9, 2019 was the day I started tracking my elastic habits with fully optimized, psychologically perfected tools. I haven't missed a day since.

Version four of the habit tracker was the winner. It worked even better than I expected, and I expected it to work well. I felt so free, so motivated, and so excited to win every day, and I won big on many days. But something special happened on August 10, 2019. That was the first day I got 100% Elite level wins. Three habits, three elite wins. A perfect day!

Early in the day, I worked out hard at the gym. Elite. Then I worked for five hours writing and editing. Elite. After that, I finished reading my 50th page of David Goggins's book, *Can't Hurt Me*. It was my third and final Elite win of the day, and I walked over to my tracker, picked up the sheet of gold stickers, and placed them all under the 10th of August.

I pounded my fist against my chest in victory. And then I realized something extraordinary. This was, coincidentally, the first day of the fourth month since I had started tracking with these updated tools, and I was more excited in this moment than I had been at any time previously. This is groundbreaking! It's not normal for this to happen in any goal or habit system. Motivation is not supposed to peak *months* into doing something; it's supposed to peak at the very beginning and then predictably and linearly wane over time as it becomes normalized. And motivation *certainly* isn't supposed to increase as neural pathways form new habits, but *mine has.*

Neuroscientists, take note. By integrating variability of result into habit formation processes, we might be able to mitigate the dreaded motivational slump as a behavior begins to transition from conscious choice to subconscious pattern. I believe we can establish a subconscious pattern of behavior ("showing up" every day) while also allowing variable choice within the pattern (lateral and vertical flexibility) to keep the conscious mind engaged. It's not different from something like gambling—the behavior is done consistently, but there is great variability within it. This stands in stark contrast to other good habit strategies that rely on behaviors done in the same way and generating the same result every time.

The elastic habits system is unlike anything I've ever experienced before. Because it's dynamic and variable, my motivation doesn't die after two weeks (as it has my whole life). My motivation still ebbs and flows with normal life circumstances, of course, but it does so at a consistently higher level now. And whenever motivation drops, I have the Mini level to keep me engaged and to keep those neural pathways firing.

When I started pounding my chest like King Kong, it hit me how special this was. I realized that every day with elastic habits is like the exciting and hopeful first day of any other goal or habit strategy. Every day of our lives is different, and finally we have a dynamic strategy to match it. Elastic habits are just as fresh and full of potential as every new day is.

Because I could easily measure and track my performance with three tiers of vertical success, I knew *exactly* how profound this day was. Since I had started my elastic habits, this was my *best day yet*. And instead of writing the same dull checkmark for months (i.e., every other habit system), I got to place three gold Elite stickers on my tracker. While the stickers are nothing more than colored paper, they are exciting. They proved that I crushed it. My super big win was immortalized in these small, symbolic circles. I even got a score bonus for it (fittingly called "Perfect Day"). You can bet I'm going to look at them again, and perhaps add some more Perfect Days to my tally.

Exciting Possibilities Are Ahead

Samuel Johnson said, "The chains of habit are too weak to be felt until they are too strong to be broken." If you want to become someone greater, you must do it with action, and not just once, but repeatedly. With time and consistency, your new habit(s) will become virtually unbreakable. It's for this reason that habit formation is among the most exciting and meaningful pursuits there is.

I'm confident that this strategy can help you stay interested, consistent, and liberated as you pursue better ways of living. In *Mini Habits*, I talked about how small steps could change your life by enabling remarkable consistency. In *Elastic Habits*, we've made our habits smarter, by letting them shrink or expand as desired or needed. We can retain all of the benefits of mini habits while gaining the excitement of bigger goal sizes. The end result is the smoothest and most satisfying way to change your life.

I think the greatest compliment you can give an author is simply to say, "I read your book." So I want to sincerely thank you for taking the time to read *Elastic Habits*. I hope this strategy improves your life as profoundly as it has improved mine. Give your habits the power of elasticity, and you will never go back to the rigid and brittle targets of the past.

Cheers,
Stephen Guise

PS. If you're interested in the custom products I've made for this system, keep reading to see how they work. Even if you don't purchase them, reading about them and seeing their design will help you to better understand how this strategy is meant to work.

ELASTIC HABIT PRODUCT MANUALS

"Seventy percent of success in life is showing up."
– Woody Allen

I've spent more than ten thousand dollars going through multiple redesigns to perfect the tools I'm about to share with you.

If you want to use items you currently have like a standard monthly calendar, I will also offer my best advice for Do-It-Yourself solutions. If you use DIY solutions instead of these official tools, just be aware they will require more maintenance since they aren't designed for this unique strategy.

These products show the strategy and tactics of *Elastic Habits*. You'll see the powerful flexibility, exciting possibilities, and seconds-per-day maintenance. Speaking of that, too many habit journals require 20 minutes of answering trite questions to "help" us do 20 minutes of work. While there are lots of options and customization involved in *Elastic Habits*, you can maintain the system in less than 20 seconds a day.

A habit strategy this impactful and unique needs a tracking system that can accommodate it. That didn't exist, so I made it. The *Elastic Habits Tracking Calendar* is customized for the strategy in this book, and it's the first product we'll look at

ELASTIC HABITS TRACKING CALENDAR

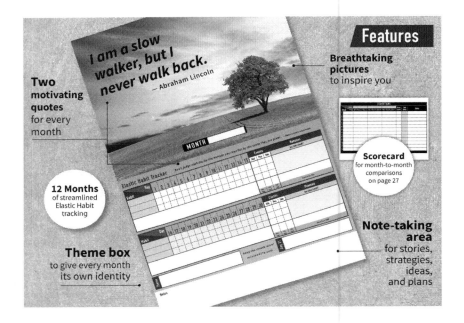

Two motivating quotes for every month

I am a slow walker, but I never walk back. — Abraham Lincoln

Features

Breathtaking pictures to inspire you

Scorecard for month-to-month comparisons on page 27

12 Months of streamlined Elastic Habit tracking

Note-taking area for stories, strategies, ideas, and plans

Theme box to give every month its own identity

Tracking is the most important part of habit formation because it fosters consistency. If your tracking system is inadequate or you don't use one, you have little chance of sustained success. Tracking is your accountability, encouragement, and momentum all in one.

The *Elastic Habits Tracking Calendar* can track three habits at a time for a full year. It's better than other habit trackers in a few ways.

1. There are *three* tiers of success, adding some much-needed variety to the habit formation process. Instead of the same check mark or X every day, you can mark the tracking calendar with color-coded stickers or symbols. If you use stickers, the color scheme is green for Mini, Silver for Plus, and Gold for Elite. No two months will be the same!

I'll reiterate what I wrote in step 6 about tracking.

> The official Elastic Habits Tracking Calendar is designed for 3/8" colored round stickers (both are sold on minihabits.com). After you complete a habit, *use the colored sticker that corresponds to the level you did* (green for Mini, silver for Plus, and gold for Elite). The stickers are the same size and shape, suggesting they are equal "wins" in many ways. Or you can use symbol progression.

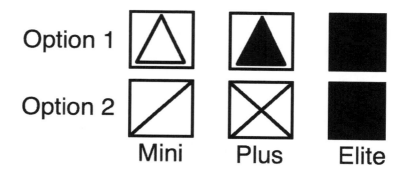

Iterative Success

If you use a marker and mark your box green for Mini, but later in the day you unexpectedly get Elite, well, your box is already green with no easy way to change it.

Using stickers, you can simply put the gold sticker *over* the green one to replace it. Similarly, the symbols above are iterative sequences that allow you to add to your current win if desired. It's important to allow for iterative upgrades in your notation because it leaves you with the opportunity to get surprise upgrade wins, which I can assure you are inspiring and delightful occurrences.

If you want to use a standard calendar, you can use stickers or symbols on the sides, top, or bottom of each day's box to correspond to your elastic habits. For example, make fitness the top left, reading the middle left, and voice training the bottom left. It's not as clean as the official tracker and lacks the scoring component, but it has the advantage of integrating into your current calendar.

It takes about 20 seconds to fill in your three habit boxes with a sticker or symbol each day. That's the only "daily maintenance" this system requires!

Objective #1 is to fill the spot. Objective #2 is to achieve higher levels. The power of elastic habits is its flexibility. If you get too focused on reaching the large goal and won't accept anything less, you're missing out on the power of flexibility. All-or-nothing thinking kills progress! If your notation is smart, it won't make one level seem vastly inferior to another, which will help you prioritize consistency, yet you will still reward yourself for bigger wins.

2. It contains two inspirational quotes and a new design every month. If you track habits on a regular calendar, the notation, look, and feel are always the same. The tracking calendar is different every month. Plus, you can start tracking your habits on *any month* (not just January).

3. It is completed 15 days at a time. When I created the first version of the Elastic Habit Tracker, it showed all

365 days of the year on one page. When I got it back from the printer, I knew I had made a mistake. It was overwhelming. The idea was to give a satisfying overview of a long winning streak. Instead, I felt stressed about having to fill in all of those blank days. One successful day felt irrelevant and small in a sea of empty spaces.

After further experimentation, I found that 15-day segments were ideal. Fifteen days was long enough to feel satisfying when completed and short enough to feel doable. Each day felt like significant progress.

With this tracking calendar, you'll be rewarded with a checkpoint every 15 days to "seal" your accomplishment and prepare for the next 15 days. You can add your 15-day scores together to get a monthly score, so you still get all the benefits of monthly tracking and month-to-month comparisons.

4. It has a scoring system. Typical habit tracking is on/off. Because our elastic habits have three levels of winning, we will have *varying* success. With the scoring system, you will know exactly how well you're doing each day, each week, and each month. Let's look at the simple scoring system.

Keeping Score

The scorecard is found on the last page of the *Elastic Habits Tracking Calendar*.

SCORECARD						
Habit				**Bonus Score**	**Total Score**	**Notes**
Month	Mini + (Plus x 2) + (Elite x 3)	Mini + (Plus x 2) + (Elite x 3)	Mini + (Plus x 2) + (Elite x 3)			
1						
2						
3						
4						
5						
6						
7						
8						
9						
10						
11						
12						

With the scorecard, you can see how each individual habit progresses from month to month, how you progress overall from month to month, and how habits compare to each other. Unlike other habit systems, this enables you to see precisely how you're doing, and *to what degree* you are succeeding.

It works as follows: Every 15 days, you count your wins at each level for each habit. Then you calculate the total points those wins are worth (Mini = 1, Plus = 2, Elite = 3). I analyzed the value of each habit, and the most obvious choice—1, 2, 3—was the best one mathematically to accurately match the value of each win. Elite habits earn 3 times as much as a Mini habit, which is significant, but three points isn't that much more than one point on an absolute level. It's a perfect balance.

But that's not all! In order to make this more fun and to help guide your perspective, there are also bonus points you can achieve.

Bonuses

Bonuses can encourage and reward you for overachievement. The most important bonus is the Habit Master bonus—it gives twice as many points as the next highest bonus! To get this bonus, all you need to do is complete the entire 15-day period without missing any habits on any day. It's named "Habit Master" because not missing days is how habits are formed and mastered. This bonus should encourage you to use the system as intended, which is to fill in tough or busy days with Mini wins instead of zeros, and do better than Mini whenever you can. Here's a list of the bonuses. These may change.

Special Achievements

- Double Down (1 Point): Meet the Elite requirement twice over in one day for one habit
- Perfect Day (2 Points): Any day with all Elite wins
- Hot Streak (3 Points): Any streak of 3+ consecutive Elite wins for one habit
- Unfreakinbelievable (5 Points): Any streak of 7+ consecutive Elite wins for one habit

15-Day Period Bonuses

- Specialist (3 Points): 10+ Elite wins for one habit this period
- Big Hitter (3 Points): 15+ total Elite wins this period
- Juggernaut (10 Points): 23+ total Elite wins this period
- Habit Master (20 Points): Zero misses this period (may use patch)

The one bonus I suggest you always use and aim for is the Habit Master bonus, because it correctly puts your focus on showing up every day. If you show up in some capacity every day, good things will happen. I promise you that. You might have days of unimpressive Mini wins, but staying in the game will give you the opportunity for huge wins later.

For something that takes just a couple of minutes to fill out, the scorecard adds a considerable amount of entertainment to the process of building life-changing habits. But it's not *just* for amusement. A standardized scoring system quantifies *exactly* how well you did for each habit, how well you did for the 15-day period, and, later, how well you did for the month. Then you can analyze your progress and make adjustments to see if you can beat your best scores. There are areas numerous places to write notes, so you can connect your scores to the different circumstances and strategies of that time in your life.

Evaluating Your Performance

If you decide to incorporate scoring, the first metric to look at, *always*, is consistency. Did you do *something* every day? Did you fill every box with a sticker or other mark of completion? If so, you've succeeded and can be very proud of your effort. It is crucial to remember this as you go along in your journey and reach higher heights. Consistency is the base of success with this strategy—once you lose that, you come undone. When skipping days becomes normal, you need to regroup.

Day 31

There are seven months with 31 days, and these days are special in the *Elastic Habits* system.

The objectives of elastic habits are freedom, autonomy, and flexibility. For all of these reasons, whenever you encounter a 31st day, it's free. By standardizing each month's tracking at 30 days (two 15-day periods), we allow for exact month-to-month comparisons and open up some fun options for that occasional extra day.

If it's the 31st day of the month, you can do whatever you want with it. This means that you can take the whole day off, but there are some other enticing options to consider. Here they are.

Day 31 Options

February Reservoir: February, the poor month, got shorted at only 28 days. Since we keep score in 15- and 30-day increments, February doesn't get a fair chance to score favorably against her 30- and 31-day siblings. If you want to bolster your February score to make it your *best month*, you can use any and all of your 31st day accomplishments toward it! Thus, if you start in March and complete every 31st day in February's honor, you'll have a whopping seven scored days to add to your February total. Lucky February then has 35 days, which is how she can go from the weakest month to the strongest!

Make-up Day: Something crazy happened on the 17th. I know. You missed a couple of habits that day. Lucky you! It's December, which has 31 days! You can use your day 31 to cover up that blemish as if it never happened. *Day 31 can substitute for any missed habit or day that month.*

Business as Usual: You may find that, even with the complete freedom to skip a full day, you want to keep your streak going. There's something special about having the ability to rest on your laurels but pushing yourself anyway. Other than adding to February's total, you don't get credit for doing day 31 that month, which is a good opportunity to prove you understand the true value of doing these beneficial behaviors (not for the score, but for yourself). The 31st is still a day, so technically, you would need to do your habits if you want to keep a days-in-a-row streak alive.

If you do take the day off and claim your 97 days-in-a-row streak on social media anyway, that's fine. It's technically not true if you skip a day 31, but within the structure of *Elastic Habits*, skipping day 31 does not invalidate your winning streak!

Free Day: After crushing it for 30 days straight, you deserve a break, right? Well, you've got one on day 31 if you want it. It's also worth noting that missing one day will never threaten your habit formation. It's missing two days in a row or frequently missing days that starts a new trend in the wrong direction. Otherwise, a single skipped day is an insignificant aberration in your sea of successful days.

I used the free day one month after three months of doing my habits every day. It was very odd. I almost had to fight myself to not do my habits. After seven months, I tried to take a free "Day 31" and still did my habits because I forgot my plan to skip them. That's the power of habit! If you take a day off, it will give you a chance to see how powerfully your habits are progressing. If you find yourself itching to get them done or even doing them without thinking, as I did, you've actually changed your brain and formed a habit!

I Missed a Habit or a Day! Now What?

Whether you miss a full day or a single habit in a single day, the *Elastic Habits* strategy offers you the opportunity for redemption. Life is crazy enough to make us miss even the easiest target (Mini) occasionally. While building winning streaks is crucial, a single miss now and again won't hurt. Just don't let it become a pattern.

One way to deal with a missed day is to use the 31st day of the month, as just discussed. If it's a 30-day month, you have another option. To deal with the occasional miss, you get one "patch" per 15-day period. This feature doesn't merely allow or encourage you to get over your mistake; *it entices you to get back on track.*

How a Patch Works

The patch is activated by writing "Patch" in the Bonuses section of your tracker. You're only allowed one per period, so be careful! The patch allows you to complete today any habits that you missed on a previous day.

If you don't use a patch, this is what it might look like if you miss a habit.

Day 9: Plus
Day 10: MISSED
Day 11: Mini
Day 12: Elite
Day 13: Plus

You have a gaping hole in your winning streak on day 10! Ack! But you can "patch it." A patch can only be applied AFTER you meet your normal habit requirements that day for the missed habit.

Example: Piano practice (Mini = 1 minute, Plus = 15 minutes, Elite = 35 minutes)

On day 11, you sit down at the piano and practice for one minute. Check! You've now completed day 11's requirement for piano. Then you remember, "Oh no, I forgot to practice Beethoven's Moonlight Sonata yesterday!" Since you've already completed day 11, you are eligible to use your patch for day 10. You practice an additional 15 minutes to earn a Plus win for the 10th. Now it looks like this.

Day 9: Plus
Day 10: Plus (Patched)

Day 11: Mini (15 extra minutes of practice today changes Day 10 to Plus win)
Day 12: Elite
Day 13: Plus

If you use a patch, you no longer have that gap.

The most valuable bonus, mentioned earlier and worth a staggering 20 points, is called Habit Master. You only get it if you don't miss a single habit in the 15-day period. It's the most lucrative bonus because nothing is more important than consistency. If you forget to do a habit and use a patch to fill the gap, it keeps you eligible for this bonus. The system rewards consistency because that's the foundation that will get you the most Elite wins in the long term!

For more on the *Elastic Habits Tracking Calendar*, such as how to use the theme box, scoring, and for video examples, visit **minihabits.com/tutorials**.

ELASTIC HABIT POSTER 2.0

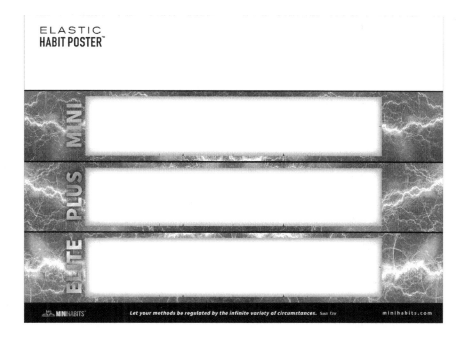

The Elastic Habit Poster 2.0 is the best way to display your elastic habits. Each poster is designed to display a single elastic habit and gives you complete flexibility to display one to eight lateral options per level. The poster is laminated for use with wet or dry erase markers.

Top Area

The top of the poster gives you ample space to describe your habit. There's enough space to turn your habit into a statement. I recommend stating your objective in a psychologically compelling way. I use the consistency template below, since that inspires me the most. I take pride in doing my most important habits *every day*.

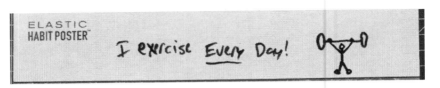

- **Identity statement:** "I am a _____!" (runner, writer, musician, etc.)
- **Consistency statement:** "I _____ every day!" (exercise, practice guitar, meditate, etc.)
- **Action description:** "_____" (reading, running, writing, etc.)

The identity statement is a powerful public declaration to yourself (and anyone else who might see the poster) that you are [a runner]. The consistency statement is a promise and declaration that you will do some amount of [running] every day. Or, if you prefer, you can simply write the action you wish to perform in the box—running, reading, healthy eating, and so on.

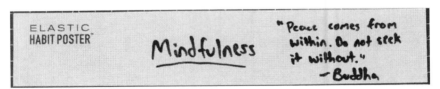

You can draw pictures. You can write quotes. You can customize it to your liking. And at the bottom of the top box, you can even label the habit columns below.

Boxes

The poster features marks on the bottom to let you design each level. I can't overstate how game-changing this is for usability! Here's how it works.

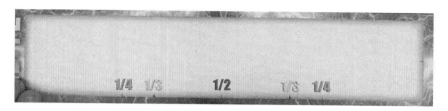

If you draw a line straight up from the small triangles at the bottom, it will create three sections (for three lateral options). Triangles have three sides, so it's intuitive. If you want two sections, simply draw a line up from the middle marker. For four sections, draw up from the middle and outer markers for exact quarter sections. On the righthand side there is an additional marker, which can bisect the box again for even more sections. And, because it's dry erase, you can always erase it and change the structure of your elastic habits.

It's important and exciting to note that this can be done with each level! That means you can have different numbers of lateral options for each vertical tier.

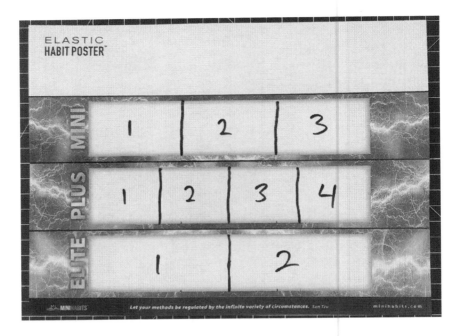

As you can see, you can completely customize your elastic habits, shaping them exactly to your preferences. Selectively narrowing and expanding vertical tiers opens up a whole new world of possibilities!

An elastic habit is clearly more advanced than the typical "do X every day" habit, but look at how simple it is to execute it. All you have to do is pick one of your options each day. It's advanced in its strategy and development of tiered options, but very simple in execution.

To give you a few ideas of what you can do, I'll show you some templates and examples.

Templates

Given the ability to increase or decrease lateral options at each level, we can powerfully guide our behavior. Let's start with the power of one. By defining just one win condition at one of the levels, we can create very interesting dynamics.

The Strong Floor Template

This template lets you define exactly where your floor is by defining only one Mini level win condition. If you set 3+ Mini win conditions, they might vary in difficulty and meaning. By having just one, you say, "This behavior at this intensity is my floor. I will always do this much or better." Then you can utilize several Plus and Elite options to entice you to do more of that behavior or others. This template is best for habits in which there is a single core behavior that must be done.

Example: Journaling

MINI	Write 1 Sentence	
PLUS	Write 1 Paragraph	Write 1 Sentence + Review 1 Week of entries
ELITE	Write 1 Page	Write 1 Paragraph + Review 1 Month of entries

Journaling is best done daily. It doesn't have to be a huge amount. It can be one sentence. But you can also review previous entries as a meaningful part of journaling. Save those for the upper level wins, some of which combine writing and reviewing.

The Silver Standard Template

This is a smart template that gives you an "assumed" moderate goal. Some people may struggle to decide between options with elastic habits, so this template gives you a single go-to option, with other options if you don't want to do the main one for any reason. Since it's at a moderate level, it shouldn't give you too much pause for being too big or too small, especially since you always have the freedom to upgrade or downgrade it as necessary.

The silver standard has just one plus-level option, and it's the option you will first aim for on any given day. Above and below it, you have easier and harder options, respectively. This way, you'll expect to get a decent win every day as a rule. If you need a break, you can move to an easier Mini win, with several options for that. And if you want to do something extra, you also have a few options for Elite wins.

Example: Exercise

MINI	3 Push-ups	10 Bodyweight Squats	2 minutes of Stretching
PLUS	Go to the gym		
ELITE	Home Workout 1 hour	Gym for 1 Hour	

If you really want to build the going-to-the-gym habit, you can set a single Plus-level goal of showing up at the gym. Then, you can set at-home exercise options at the Mini level, for days you can't make it for whatever reason. And set a few stretch goals for once you arrive at the gym—such as time exercised, specific workout programs, or even home workouts (which can be just as intense as the gym).

The White Whale Template

In *Moby Dick*, the sailor Ahab is obsessed with hunting a massive white whale named Moby Dick. From this story has come the concept of your "white whale," that one thing that you must conquer, even though the challenge seems insurmountable at times. With the White Whale Template, you only have one Elite target. It is your white whale. If you are going to earn this level, it's going to be this one thing. Nothing else can match it.

To help you in your quest to slay that Elite whale as often as you can, you'll have several Plus and Mini options for support. These are still valuable parts of your journey, but this template really puts the spotlight on that whale! And really, that's what these one-win strategies do—they emphasize a single behavior as very important.

This one is fun because it makes the Elite level stand apart as extra special and exciting, kind of like a massive white whale!

Example: Healthy Eating

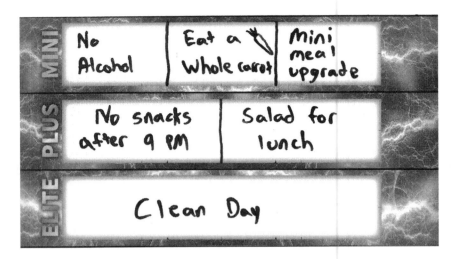

There are a number of ways you could do this, depending on your approach and goals. In this example, Elite victory is gained with a "clean day," defined as no added sugar, processed foods, or alcohol consumed. And then you can have several Plus and Mini goals with smaller accomplishments to aim for.

Those are the one-win templates. You can even have one win condition in two levels. Maybe you have one condition for Mini and Elite and a few Plus options in the middle for flexibility, as in this example below.

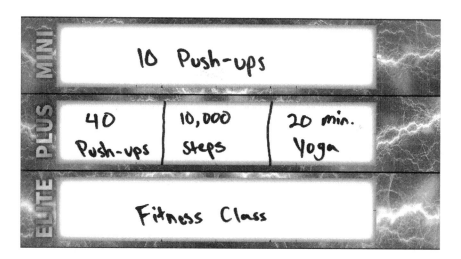

The Habit Pool Template

The idea with habit pools is to not tie behaviors to any level, but instead add a group of moderate-easy behaviors into a giant pool. If you complete one, it's Mini, two is Plus, and any three is Elite. To do this with the poster, I recommend using a different color marker to visually differentiate a habit pool habit from your other elastic habits. And you can also label it in the upper box.

Example: Exercise Habit Pool

MINI	Treadmill 10 min.	Yoga 15 min.	25 Push-ups
PLUS	20 Bodyweight Squats	15 Pull-ups	40 Sit-ups
ELITE	50 Jumping Jacks	Dance to 3 Songs	Walk 5,000 Steps

A habit pool ignores levels. Do any one of these for Mini, any two for Plus, and any three for Elite. If you want to make it really interesting, you can pool part of your habit. For example, maybe you have one Elite option of going to the gym, but make Mini and Plus a pool where one gets Mini and any two gets Plus (but for Elite, you must get to the gym).

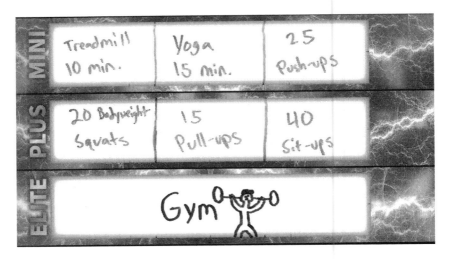

What? No, the bar is going BEHIND his head.

Further Notes

This is the best habit system in the world. Not only can your habits adapt to you every single day, but you can design them with your specific lifestyle in mind. The options are limitless.

In some cases, it's useful to *limit* the verticality of a lateral option. For me, going to the gym is always an Elite level victory. Whenever I go to the gym, I always work out intensely, so it doesn't make sense for me to have lower-level options for the gym. But that's specific to my behavior when I arrive at the gym.

On the other side of the spectrum, I could set a Mini-level-only win condition of buying a new book for my reading habit. Buying interesting books is an essential part of the reading process that involves some research, and yet, I'm certainly not going to give myself a Plus or Elite level win for buying more books. It would only make sense to give myself Mini level credit for taking that small step to purchase something to read, because researching and buying a book to read is about the same difficulty as reading two pages of a book (my other Mini win condition).

Don't feel that when you create a win condition, it must be adapted to all three levels. Only do that when it makes sense and benefits you!

Habit Design Quick Guide

With so many options for habit design with the Habit Poster 2.0, how do you choose what to do?

1. Start with a broad habit. What do you want to do? Exercise? Read? Write? Journal? Clean your home? Organize your digital life? Start a hobby? Learn a new skill?

2. Determine the end goal. What is this habit going to accomplish for you? Where do you want to go with it? What's the ideal outcome?

3. Based on responses to the first two questions, list the fundamental and supplementary tasks of the habit. Fundamental tasks are the only ones you should use for any of the single-win condition templates we discussed earlier. They work well alone because they are fundamental to the habit and are therefore worthy of the spotlight. Supplementary tasks have value, and may even be necessary for the habit in smaller doses, but they aren't useful as your primary focus.

For playing guitar, practicing with your fingers is fundamental. You can read every guitar lesson book in the world, but if you don't practice it with your own hands, you won't be able to do it! Music theory and things like that could be considered supplementary tasks.

For exercise, you might determine that aerobic training is fundamental if your goal is heart health and weight management. Or maybe weightlifting is your fundamental goal for strength and body-building. Then other forms of exercise could supplement that. Or you might want well-rounded fitness—in which case a large number of exercise options are fundamentally relevant to your goal.

If a task is supplementary, try to pair it with other supplementary tasks at whatever level(s) you place it. Give yourself options. You can also pair fundamental and supplementary tasks together. But these are guidelines more than rules. You might put a supplementary task as your only Mini win condition just to make sure it gets done to some degree, and then focus on your fundamental tasks at the Plus and Elite levels.

4. With your list of behaviors, decide your win conditions, one at a time. Start with the Mini level and choose what behavior(s) at what intensity will earn you a Mini win. Then move to Plus and Elite. Alternatively, choose one of the templates discussed earlier and see if it works with your habit. The ideal structure of your elastic habit will depend on your specific goals for the habit.

I understand this can seem overwhelming because of the literally infinite possibilities of elastic habit design, but let me clarify how easy this is. If you want, you can set one win condition for each level. That's the simplest elastic habit and it can work very well. I recommend starting simply and building from there. Don't add extra options just because you think you "should."

If it's been a month and you've never done one of your options, consider removing or revising it. Dead weight in the form of unused options won't help much.

Finally, don't feel like you need to figure everything out at the very beginning. These posters are dry erase. Use your eraser as much as you want to restructure your habits to work for you. This isn't a cookie-cutter method, because *you can customize it to your exact goals and your exact life.* That's why it's going to work better than anything else you've ever tried. Once you optimize it, you're going to wonder why you didn't have this sooner.

It will take some time to figure out what works best. And you will get new ideas as you go. But it's a very fun process and it never gets stale, because elastic habits can change themselves as much as they change you (significantly!).

You can buy these posters at minihabits.com. If you prefer to do it yourself, you can simply use a whiteboard. The posters have some advantages over the whiteboard, such as the perfect division marks and the fact that they're specifically designed for this.

INTERACTIVE HABIT POSTER
(LIMITED EDITION)

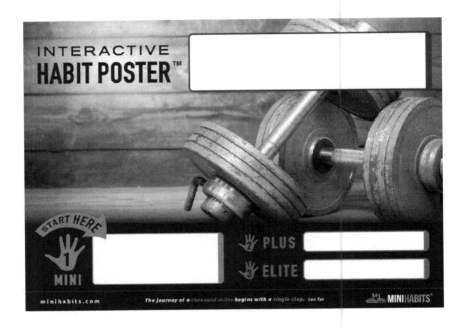

Interactive Habit Posters are used to display one elastic habit. They sacrifice the flexibility of the Elastic Habit Poster 2.0 for style. You have less room to write your options, and in return, get a large, beautiful picture to represent your habit.

There are 25 different themes. These posters are laminated for wet and dry erase marker usage, allowing you to edit your poster as much as you want.

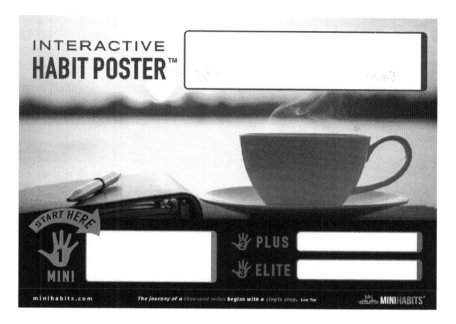

You can fill in your lateral and vertical options in the Mini, Plus, and Elite boxes. Review Part Five if you don't yet know your vertical and lateral options.

Once you've filled in your poster, put it on the wall in a place you'll see every day. If you have a "command center" where you organize your life, that's the right place. For me, that's in the bedroom. For others, it might be near their desk or on the refrigerator with their calendar. I bought a giant magnetic whiteboard to display my habit posters, tracker, and any other daily to-dos or notes.

I recommend the Habit Poster 2.0 in general over these, but Interactive Habit Posters work well for simple habits and for those who want to try out slap contracts (covered next).

Slap Contracts

People are generally more successful at showing up to work than they are at pursuing personal goals. We adhere to the work contract—we show up, work, and we get paid for it. Why is it any different with personal goals?

You are the arbitrator. When it comes to your personal goals, you can *always* break your agreement as if it never existed. Even if you set up a punishment for non-compliance, you can then break *that contract.* No matter what you do, you have the freedom to not comply without direct consequences. You are the all-powerful arbitrator in your personal life, and you know it.

Given our personal power to cancel pursuits on a whim, it's a challenge to do beneficial things that we resist doing. We often try to set up a sort of boss/employee relationship to ensure our success, but in the long run, we still change our minds and do what we want.

To fix this, you can create a likable arbitrator to hand your executive power to temporarily. That arbitrator is your habit poster, and the way to make deals using it is through slap contracts.

Slap contracts are optional, and in practice, I find myself interacting with my posters this way only about 10–20% of the time. It's a nice option to have when you're on the fence and want to commit to doing something.

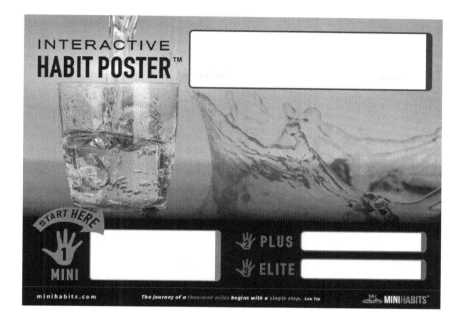

How the Slap Contract Works

Once two parties sign a written contract, it's official and *legally binding*. It becomes real, strong, and formidable. Wouldn't it be great if powerful words like that could describe our commitment to our goals?

A slap contract is a simple gesture that signals your absolute intention to take a particular action right now. Like written contracts, a slap contract is meant to be serious and binding, but it's a contract with yourself. In practice, it's done by simply touching (or lightly slapping) the habit poster on your wall. I'm aware that it sounds silly, but you've got to try it!

Here's how it works: By making contact with the poster, be it a slap, "bro fist," flick, or any other kind of touch, you declare your intention. Each "slap" of the poster commits you to the next highest level.

1 slap: Mini level
2 slaps: Plus level
3 slaps: Elite level

You can also slap the poster *after* you complete an action to celebrate. Disclaimer: I am not responsible for any damage caused from slapping your poster too emphatically. Slap at your own risk! Use this technique to solidify your intention and make it tangible. It's a lot stronger than simply thinking about doing the behavior.

My Slap Story: I had been crushing my habits lately, hitting the Elite level consistently on multiple habits, and I found out that one of my favorite video game series had a Japanese-only game that had been translated to English. So I excitedly thought, "I've been doing well, I'm going to take a break. I'll make this a Mini-level day so I can play this game."

I read a mere three pages of *On Writing* by William Zinsser to satisfy my two-pages reading requirement. You can slap the poster beforehand to declare your intention **or** you can slap it afterwards to celebrate its completion. I was excited to have met my requirement so easily and eager to play the game. In my excitement, I quickly slapped the poster *twice* to celebrate my easy win. Twice? Oops! That meant I had to read the rest of the chapter (because two slaps is a Plus level commitment, which means reading at least one chapter).

I found the situation amusing because it "forced" me to read a little bit more than I normally would have, but it was my own doing, so I couldn't complain. Poster interactions always feel fair. If you don't want to be on the hook for the action, you simply don't touch the poster. If you do touch it, then you must follow through.

Poster Interaction

I recommend that you only create a slap contract the instant before you begin to execute it. When your hand contacts the poster, your very next step needs to be in the direction of that action. No skipping. No excuses. You must do it after that. It's best done this way to preserve your trust in the process.

If it's running, get your shoes on in the next minute and walk out the door. If you touch that poster, you are on the hook. You'll find that it's more empowering than draining to make a self-contract. I find that it's comforting in a way to know that the action will be done when I activate a contract. It removes any doubt and ambiguity that I might not show up. If you make your contract too early and something affects your ability to execute, you may lose trust in it.

Slap contracts are not confining or restrictive because they're completely choice-driven. *You* are the one who activates the contract. It's not from a goal you set two months ago. It's not a part of a rigid program you're following to get ripped abs "in only 7 days." It's you. In the same way that I accept all of the contracts I've signed for my books, you'll accept these contracts because *you* activate them. If you don't want to do the action, don't activate the contract. It's that simple. And since these contracts will be optional, you'll never have guilt, shame, or paralyzing pressure about (not) doing them.

The Importance of the "Handshake"

As many others have written before, it can help to write down your intentions somewhere—on a white board, on your calendar, etc. Slap contracts take this concept to another level, and here's why.

Writing something down on a board MIGHT be enough to set your intention, but you still have to take a few steps to "seal" that intention. Why? *We've all written things down and not done them.* That reduces our trust that writing something down means it will absolutely be done. That's nothing close to a legally binding contract. The other issue is that writing something down doesn't mean anything unless we consciously note that writing "Read a page in a book" on the whiteboard means that we intend to do it. We still have to assign meaning to the words.

This is an opportunity to create more powerful intentions. You will see the poster and know what it offers. Your brain will know exactly what it means when you touch or enthusiastically slap the poster. You're in. You're doing it.

Contract Troll (Toll)

There's one more way to use a habit poster—as a contract troll.

The contract troll gets its name from the classic story of the troll on the bridge, requiring a toll for people to pass. I have a pull-up bar in my bathroom doorway (the bar prevents the door from closing, but I live alone, so I don't need to close the door); every time I leave the restroom, I require myself to pay a "toll" of at least two pull-ups (or substitute five push-ups). I require it when I'm leaving as opposed to entering because if I have to use the restroom, I don't want to have to do pull-ups first.

Consider setting up small "tolls" for certain actions in key places. Exercise is a likely application—push-ups or pull-ups—but there are other creative ideas. For example, maybe you require yourself to have a "shot" of water every time you open the fridge or enter the kitchen. Have a small water glass nearby, and then quickly fill it up and drink it. That's an easy way to increase your water intake.

THE HABIT STAR

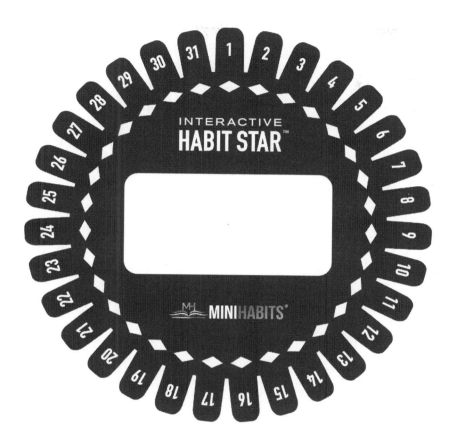

The Habit Star is a fun and versatile habit tracker. It's separate from the core *Elastic Habits* system; it fills other habit tracking needs.

The Habit Star has 31 numbered tabs centered on a circular base. The tabs fold back, which represents completion of that number or day. The tabs will stay back if the center of the star is affixed to the wall and/or by placing small Velcro stickers to the tabs (I sell these, too). When a tab is folded behind, the green back side can be seen through a diamond-shaped cutout, which gives a visually satisfying "success" mark.

As for what to put in the box, you have several options. You can draw a baby dinosaur to represent your paleontology studies. You can make it cryptic if it relates to a bad habit you don't want to advertise (My Habit Star says "freedom" to represent what I'll gain by abstaining from a bad habit).

Five Ways to Use a Habit Star

1. Track a behavior for the month.
Every month has 31 days or fewer. Thus, each numbered tab represents one day of the month. If you make it all the way through day 31 without missing a day, your star will become a cool-looking circle!

You can track good or bad habits this way. For good habits, fold down the tab for any successful day. It's important to note that the Habit Star lacks vertical flexibility, so try to use it for on/off habits such as brushing your teeth or flossing that have a low "ceiling" but are still important.

For bad habits, fold down a tab for each day that you do NOT do the bad habit. Since the tabs are green and denote success, you want to associate folding them down with doing the right thing. It's really satisfying!

Did you go a full day without eating added sugar? Put the tab down! Other bad habits you could target with the Habit Star are biting your nails, eating out, smoking, drinking, or spending more than two hours on social media. Your options are endless, and because the Habit Star is interactive and visual, you'll feel greater satisfaction as you break bad habits.

Each morning, I get up and think about yesterday. If I succeeded in avoiding my bad habit, I put the next tab down. You can just as well do it for good habits. If I did the bad habit, I can either leave the tab up or try to start over with a new streak. Whether you start over or not depends on your goals. Breaking bad habits can be difficult, so you might go into it with the perspective of seeing how many days out of the month you can win (allowing for mistakes) instead of letting one mistake derail you.

Alternatively, mark the tab down before the day begins as a precommitment. If you succeed, leave it down. If you don't, flip it back (this is additional motivation to stick with it!).

2. Track a streak (good or bad habit), starting whenever.

You don't have to use the start of a month to start a streak with the #1 tab. Make any day your "day one" of a new behavior pattern. This is my preferred use of the habit star, and, specifically, I like to use it for keeping tabs on bad habits since I use the *Elastic Habits* system for good habits. If it's already the 16th of the month, you can start tracking on that day.

3. Track on/off days for a behavior, starting whenever or monthly.

There are some behaviors, such as eating certain foods or drinking alcohol, that you might not want to cut out of your life completely, but moderate instead. Or maybe it's a behavior that you do want to eliminate eventually, but not immediately. For a bad behavior that you want to limit, put the tab down on days you succeed, and leave them up on ones you don't. At the end of the 31 days, you'll see exactly how many times you did (not) do that behavior.

This works with good habits as well. Target behaviors that

you don't want or need to do every day, but that are great when you can do them. For me, that would be eating "mega salads." They are superbly healthy, but I don't want to require that I have one every day. Still, I might want to encourage myself to make them more frequently, and tracking them on a Habit Star can encourage that. Also, my dentist wants me to floss more. But I personally don't think it needs to be done daily, so I can track the days I do it with a Habit Star.

4. Count reps and "laps" (day).
Next to my pull-up bar, I have a Habit Star on the wall. I like to do pull-ups throughout the day sometimes, and instead of keeping track in my head, I can use the Habit Star to keep count.

Here's how it works: if I start off with a set of eight pull-ups, I put down the #8 tab. Later, if I do four more, I'll pull the #8 tab back up and flip down the #12 tab. Once I make it around the star, I'll keep the #1 tab down to remind myself that I've completed "one lap" around the star. It's really fun and encourages me to do more than I would otherwise. Sometimes I go for 100 reps, which is three laps around the star (93 reps) plus seven more.

5. Count reps (week or month).
Maybe you want to eat more carrots, but you don't necessarily want to demand that you do it every day. You might eat three carrots on one day, and none the next. In this case, you might want to count how many (full-size) carrots you eat in a month (or week or any amount of time you desire). As with the pull-ups, simply flip the tab that currently represents the number of carrots you've eaten in total. In this case, you won't reset the count at the end of the day; you'll keep the count for the entire week or month or whatever period of time you deem best.

When you flip a tab down, the number is no longer visible, but you can easily tell what number you're at by looking at the surrounding numbers. Or simply flip the Habit Star over and you'll see all of the folded-down numbers.

Conclusion and DIY Idea

The Habit Star can track or count anything. Best of all, it's reusable. After each period of 31 days, you can mark that you've completed one month and reset the star for the next one.

If you want to try a DIY solution, I can tell you that the idea for this product came from posters with the phone number tabs you can pull off. You know, the ones you see on electrical poles? You could cut a piece of paper into 31 tabs, number them, and tear them off as you complete them. It won't look as pretty as the Habit Star and won't be reusable, and you'd have to write 1– 31 each time, but it could still be worthwhile!

If you're interested to see a demonstration of the Habit Star, visit **minihabits.com**.

Thank You

Thank you for reading *Elastic Habits*! If you want to know more about the tools and strategy, visit **minihabits.com** for supplementary materials.

If you believe this book shares an important message, please leave a review. Reviews are the main metric people use to judge a book's content. If you make progress, please come back and tell other readers (and me) about it!

Every single review has a huge impact on others' willingness to read a book, and if this strategy changes your life, you can change someone else's life by spreading the word. The impact and reach of this book is up to you. *Mini Habits* is proof of this. Because readers have reviewed and shared it, it is now read all over the world! Will you help me spread the message of *Elastic Habits*? The world needs to hear it.

Other Books by Stephen Guise

Mini Habits
Although you don't need to read *Mini Habits* to benefit from *Elastic Habits*, it will show you the nuts and bolts of the original strategy that changed lives and ultimately inspired this strategy.

Book: amazon.com/dp/B00HGKNBDK
Video Course: udemy.com/course/mini-habit-mastery/

Mini Habits for Weight Loss
Diets have been shown to make you gain weight, even more than not dieting. Instead, try this habit-driven approach to weight loss, and your changes can last.

Book: amazon.com/dp/B01N0FR4AX
Video Course: udemy.com/course/weight-loss-mini-habits/

How to Be an Imperfectionist (Book)
This book applies *Mini Habits* to the problem of perfectionism. If you struggle with depression, fear, and inaction, this book has a lot to offer.

Book: amazon.com/dp/B00UMG535Y

Tuesday Messages
Every Tuesday, I write to subscribers. People have told me this content is life-changing.
Sign up: stephenguise.com/subscribe/

Introduction

1   A caveat: When you stop exercising completely after doing it consistently, you can see all of the benefits that it was giving you. After this experience, I was admittedly eager to get active again. For that reason, and the fact that those exercise neural pathways still existed in my brain, it wasn't a perfect scientific experiment. But it did put me into a familiar place—I desperately wanted to get back in shape and had the potential to do so, yet felt completely hopeless about it.

2   A Closer Look at How Vultures Lazily Circle in the Air (2019). https://www.audubon.org/news/a-closer-look-how-vultures-lazily-circle-air-1

3   Fun fact: Hang gliders are unpowered winged aircraft that launch from tow planes or the tops of mountains. They then glide down to ground level. But an expert glider can use updrafts to gain elevation, remain airborne, and even travel! The world record cross-country hang glider flight lasted 24 hours. That's an incredible feat considering that it's a stationary glider with no motor (and no public restroom). That's the power of updrafts!

Chapter 1

1   Instead of swimming butterfly into the strength of a rip current, you can swim breaststroke (the easiest stroke) or freestyle (a faster and less tiring stroke than butterfly) parallel to the shore to exit the current. With greater knowledge of how riptides (and swimming) work, you can make much better decisions if you are caught in one.

2   There's an important caveat to this that you might be thinking about. There are times when a mindless and forced "just take action" stance is beneficial or best for a situation. The *Elastic Habits* strategy provides a vehicle for self-forced action called "slap contracts"—we'll talk about those at the end of the book, and no, they don't involve physical violence.

Chapter 2

1   Discipline vs. Self-Discipline, what's the difference? (2019). https://medium.com/@CMAHCA/discipline-vs-self-discipline-whats-the-difference-3371ada3151e

2   Patrick Henry's "Liberty or Death" Speech (2019). Retrieved from https://www.history.com/news/patrick-henrys-liberty-or-death-speech-240-years-ago

Chapter 3

1   I briefly considered naming this book "Plastic Habits," as it has interesting connotations with brain plasticity *and* physics plasticity, but I feared "plastic habits" would make people think this book was about habitually littering or recycling plastic. So instead, I went with a title that makes people think of yoga pants. Ah, much better.

2   Fun fact: According to the United States Library of Congress, the deepest

tree roots come from a wild fig tree in South Africa. Its root system was found to reach 400 feet deep! That's equivalent in height to a 37-story building. Source: Tree Planting - Interesting Tree Facts - United Nations Environment Programme (2019). http://webarchive.loc.gov/all/20050723150643/http://www.unep.org/documents.multilingual/default.asp?DocumentID=445&ArticleID=4852&l=en

Chapter 4

[1] In case you don't know, a planche push-up looks like someone doing a push-up on the moon—their feet remain off the ground as they push up! And somehow, people do it with full Earthen physics in play.

[2] Shugart, C. (2019). All Muscle, No Iron. T Nation. Retrieved from https://www.t-nation.com/training/all-muscle-no-iron

[3] Shugart, C. ibid.

[4] *Mini Habits* did have a small amount of vertical flexibility built-in in the form of "bonus reps," but they were undefined and undeveloped.

[5] Huang, S., Jin, L., & Zhang, Y. (2017). Step by step: Sub-goals as a source of motivation. *Organizational Behavior and Human Decision Processes*, 141, 1–15. doi: 10.1016/j.obhdp.2017.05.001

Chapter 5

[1] Man tries to kiss snake, then gets bitten (2019). Retrieved from https://www.bbc.com/news/world-us-canada-39956904

Chapter 7

[1] Sun Tzu. The Art of War (2015) (Chiron Academic Press – The Original Authoritative Edition) (pp. 40-41). Wisehouse. Kindle Edition.

[2] Sun Tzu. ibid. (p. 40).

[3] Sun Tzu. ibid. (p. 41).

Chapter 8

[1] Schwartz, B. The Paradox of Choice [Video]. Retrieved from https://www.ted.com/talks/barry_schwartz_on_the_paradox_of_choice?language=en

[2] Group, E. (2019). EWG's 2019 Shopper's Guide to Pesticides in Produce™. Retrieved from https://www.ewg.org/foodnews/summary.php

Chapter 9

[1] Blumenthal, J., Smith, P., & Hoffman, B. (2012). Is exercise a viable treatment for depression?. Retrieved from https://www.ncbi.nlm.nih.gov/pmc/articles/PMC3674785/

[2] The diaphragm is a muscle involved in breathing, speaking, and singing. It

can be very useful to strengthen it. Cleveland Clinic has a handy guide for how to exercise your diaphragm, if you're interested.

Chapter 10

[1]   I hope one day I can become a world-class skier and make this anecdote more impressive in retrospect. Look for my next book, *How I Became the Triple Black Diamond Champion of the World*. That probably won't happen, because I still kind of hate snow skiing (water skiing is great fun!). Even after my braking breakthrough, one especially sharp, steep turn would still force me to pancake myself into the snow (instead of a tree). Turning would have been my next breakthrough!